# TALKING FAT

## Health vs. Persuasion in the War On Our Bodies

### Lonie McMichael, Ph.D.

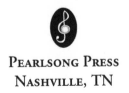

PEARLSONG PRESS
NASHVILLE, TN

Pearlsong Press
P.O. Box 58065
Nashville, TN 37205
www.pearlsong.com
www.pearlsongpress.com

Trade paperback ISBN: 9781597190633
Ebook ISBN: 9781597190640

Book & cover design by Zelda Pudding.

Health At Every Size® and HAES℠ are registered trademarks and service marks of the Association for Size Diversity and Health (www.sizediversityandhealth.org) and are used with permission. Spelling and word usage in blog posts and the preferred noncapitalization of some names has been preserved in quotes and references in this book, with the exception of the occasional correction of apparent typos.

Library of Congress Cataloging-in-Publication Data

McMichael, Lonie, 1966–
 Talking fat : health vs. persuasion in the war on our bodies / Lonie McMichael.
    p. cm.
Includes bibliographical references.
ISBN 978-1-59719-063-3 (original trade pbk. : alk. paper)—ISBN 978-1-59719-064-0 (ebook)
 1. Obesity—Health aspects. 2. Obesity—Social aspects. 3. Health behavior. 4. Communication in medicine. I. Title.
RA645.O23M38 2012
616.3'98—dc23

                                    2012017446

To my mother, Rose Cobb,
who always believed in me,
and
to my partner, Tully Dozier,
for supporting me every step of the way.

# Contents

# Acknowledgements

This book would never have made it to print without the help and influence of a number of people. My dissertation chair, Dr. Amy Koerber, supported and encouraged me throughout the research and writing process, giving me excellent feedback and challenging me in many positive ways. My partner, Tully Dozier, has listened to me rage, cry, and crow throughout the process of bringing this book to fruition—supporting me and telling me I could do it, over and over again. Thank you both for your belief in me above all else.

I also want to thank the incredible women and men of the Fatosphere, fat studies, and the fat acceptance movement. They taught me, they guided me, they supported me, they shared their lives with me—often never knowing how much their gifts of sharing their stories and viewpoints helped me grow. They show me bravery and strength every day—whether it be just in living the best life they can, in their determination to love themselves, or in being wild and wonderful fat activists. These people are my heroes.

# CHAPTER 1
## It's Not About Health

Sarah Watson decided to become a triathlete—a laudable goal for anyone. Sarah was fat. Yet she succeeded.

She trained, she ran, she swam, and she biked. She participated in at least seven triathlons; she came in toward the last, but she finished. She decided to post her experiences on a blog—not to be anyone's hero, but to show that a person could be fat and fit. When Kate Harding's "Illustrated BMI Project"—an online slideshow presenting individuals of different sizes, designed "to demonstrate just how ridiculous the BMI standards are"—came out, Sarah was originally pictured in a swimsuit at a swim meet. In response, Sarah received numerous attacking comments left at her blog. Based on that single picture, assumptions were made about her body including that she was

> unhealthy, weak, sick, in need of medical attention, grinding my joints to a pulp, not an athlete, not a triathlete, lying about what I eat (which I never discuss online), lying about the levels of exercise I do (which I also don't discuss in intimate detail), self-hating, and a whole host of other things.

Sarah decided to take down her blog, a decision she explained in a guest post at Kate Harding's *Shapely Prose* blog:

> I went and exercised. I had fun. I exercised for three years and then decided to do something a little unusual. I did a triathlon. And I liked it so much, I did seven more in one year. And wrote about it. And posted pictures. And talked about how I felt. And talked about how others made me feel. And talked about it from the perspective of the fat chick who's usually last. And talked about the fun I had. And talked about the bad things. And I didn't hold back.
>
> Somehow, that became permission for every asshat on the web to dissect my entire life based on a picture or reading one or two blog entries.

Sarah did go back to blogging a few weeks later after changing her comments policy to reduce the number of what bloggers call "trolls," which the *Urban Dictionary* defines as a "depraved individual who sits in front of a computer all day and posts flames of an idiotic or pseudo-intellectual nature on public forums and private websites." However, she stopped blogging completely a few months later. I do not know if she is still training or participating in triathlons.

As Sarah's story reveals, fat prejudice is thriving in American society today. Even when trying to "get healthy," to live by society's rules, fat individuals still face ridicule and prejudice in everyday life—ridicule and prejudice that have not been censured by society.

Why do we allow such prejudice to persist, when as a society we usually condemn prejudice? We allow such prejudice to exist based upon two faulty premises: that fat people are fat because they eat too much and exercise too little, and that fat in and of itself is unhealthy. In this book I show the faulty science behind these two premises and the problems such beliefs have caused.

WE ARE AT WAR WITH FAT PEOPLE IN THIS COUNTRY. IT IS a war that is proclaimed with as much righteousness as the Crusades. It is a justified war, because, you see, we are only trying to save people from themselves. We are only trying to make people HEALTHY. We are trying to cajole, shame, encourage and, if necessary, force them to fit an unrealistic norm—but that's OK, because it's for their own good.

And it is a war built on a lie—the lie that the war is about health.

The *last* thing the war on the "obesity epidemic" is about is health, which I show throughout this book. I examine what the war is really about by looking at the rhetoric—the persuasion endemic to the assault.

The "obesity epidemic" is about many, many things—prejudice, money, scapegoats, etc.—but what it isn't about is health. It's a war on everyday people. And it isn't making anyone healthier.

## *Background of the Project*

IN THE FALL OF 2003 I STARTED WORKING TOWARD MY MASter's degree in technical communication at Texas State University. At the same time, after thirty years of failing at diets, I started exploring body and fat acceptance. Throughout gaining a master's and Ph.D. in technical communication, I explored the fat experience. Seeing the part that medical rhetoric is playing in the oppression of fat individuals, I decided to write my dissertation using bell hooks' theories of oppression to examine our ideas of fat within the United States.

The result was a work with two distinct sections: one examining the medical rhetoric surrounding the "obesity epidemic" and focusing on the idea of normalization, and the other using hooks' theories to explore fat prejudice. *Talking Fat* focuses on the first part of the project. Another book will contain the work on fat prejudice: *Acceptable Prejudice? Fat and Social Justice in the U.S.*

A number of research projects have added to the content of *Talking Fat*. Throughout the process of researching and writing I explored the medical literature surrounding "obesity" and the "obesity epidemic," as well as literature that falls into the fat studies or fat acceptance arena. Prior to beginning the dissertation research, I had already conducted three limited research projects using hooks' ideology in terms of fat:

- A textual analysis of blogs conducted in the fall of 2006. In this project I considered more than fifty actual postings from online fat-centered communities collectively known as the Fatosphere, such as *Big Fat Blog, Shapely Prose,* and *The Rotund.*

- An online focus group conducted in the spring of 2007 that spotlighted internalization and resistance processes in light of bell hooks' ideology of domination.

- A mini-study of medical articles in the fall of 2007 in which I examined a few medical study reports published in leading medical journals and responses to those articles in order to better understand medical findings and the medical community's attitudes toward fat.

My final and largest project had two distinct parts: a series of email interviews with Fatosphere participants and a rhetorical analysis—using bell hooks' ideology of domination as a lens— of blog posts in the Fatosphere. Through these examinations of the lives of fat people—fat people who no longer believe they are "bad" for being fat—*Talking Fat* and *Acceptable Prejudice?* have come to be.

I thought long and hard about writing *Talking Fat*. I am NOT a scientist, nor will I claim to have scientific knowledge. Yet I am an expert in how we talk about science and health and the greater implications of such conversations. I am also an expert in research methods. By the very nature of this project

I have to approach the science and the research, understanding the rhetoric behind it. That I don't have explicit medical training may be valuable. In the process of learning their fields, scientists and medical professionals are indoctrinated into a particular way of thinking—a way of thinking that I have not adopted. So by looking from the outside in, I can provide an alternative way of thinking about the science surrounding fat.

Studying the "obesity epidemic," medicine surrounding fat, and fat acceptance has broadened my viewpoint. I have chosen to write this book not only as a scholar, but as an individual who has experienced fat prejudice and fat hate the majority of my life. I named the book *Talking Fat* not just because I'm looking at how we talk about fat, but as a voice for the fat individual—people who often experience being silenced in many, many ways. I hope that, as I balance those two roles—the scholar and the fat person—I will help you understand the part that fat plays in your own life, your own attitudes, and our society as a whole.

# *Terms, Entities & Expressions*

THROUGHOUT THIS WORK I USE WORDS AND PHRASES THAT may not be known to you or language that might confuse you. This section explains terms you may not be familiar with or may not have heard before, and my reasoning behind using the language as I do.

## *Fat Positive Entities*

I AM PRO-FAT. THAT DOES NOT MEAN I WANT EVERYONE TO BE fat, nor does it mean that I want everyone to sit around watching TV and eating bonbons *(yecch!)*. What it does mean is that I believe that fat people deserve to be treated like people—that fat people deserve to have the same rights, options and attention as other people in society. This revolutionary belief comes out of the fat acceptance movement.

According to Esther Rothblum and Sandra Solovay in *The Fat Studies Reader*, the fat acceptance movement is a grassroots movement that has its origins in U.S. feminism of the 1970s. To understand the ideas presented in this movement, we must first have an idea of what "fat acceptance" means and the basic tenets of that philosophy.

Fat acceptance appears to be exactly that: the acceptance of fat by cultures around the world (in the framework of this book, specifically the dominant culture of the U.S. as a whole). The fat acceptance movement is the cornerstone of resistance to the current dominant ideals regarding fat. Rothblum and Solovay note that this movement has also been called the "fat liberation movement," with members being referred to as the "fat pride community" by fat activists such as the indomitable Marilyn Wann. In fact, a segment of the movement would like to focus on fat pride rather than fat acceptance—to learn to be proud of the fat body, not just accept it.

The movement is exemplified by the National Association to Advance Fat Acceptance (NAAFA), which was founded in 1969. NAAFA is a civil rights organization "dedicated to ending size discrimination in all of its forms," says their website. The Association for Size Diversity and Health (ASDAH) is also associated with the fat acceptance movement. ASDAH promotes Health At Every Size® (HAES$^{SM}$), a weight-neutral approach to health that respects diversity in body size. In the summer of 2011, ASDAH trademarked the term "Health At Every Size" in an attempt to keep it from being co-opted in support of dieting.

The fat acceptance movement has resurged and expanded greatly in the last decade, thanks to the advent of the World Wide Web and the pressure to eliminate fat in our society. The primary space of fat acceptance online is currently called the Fatosphere—a loosely connected online community of resistance made up of blog spaces and other social media and populated by fat acceptance advocates. Blogger Kate Harding credits FatFu, another fat acceptance blogger, for popularizing the term "Fatosphere" when she founded the "Notes from the Fatosphere" RSS feed in May 2007, according to Fatosphere participant Meowser.

At first *Big Fat Blog* was the only fat acceptance blog actively discussing such concepts, but in 2007 Marianne Kirby of *The Rotund* and Kate Harding of *Shapely Prose* both joined in. By the end of that year, with the addition of a number of fat acceptance blogs the Fatosphere had become an entity, according to Harding and Kirby in their book *Lesssons from the Fatosphere*.

The Fatosphere community is made up of a variety of views on fat acceptance,. As Harding and Kirby point out, "it's a smorgasbord of different takes on fat acceptance, body image, sexuality, disability and self-esteem." Individuals often connect to the Fatosphere through one of three RSS feeds. "Notes from the Fatosphere" and the "Fat Chat Feed" are both administered by the Australian academician and fat activist Bri King. They basically contain the same information, though King says the "Notes" feed has a few more blogs.

King gives guidelines for acceptable blogs for the "Notes" feed:

* Your blog posts are primarily related to fat, that is fat commentary, fat fashion, living fat, fat and health/health professions, HAES or the like. Your submission will not be accepted if your blog entries are not at least 75% relating to fat/size acceptance—Notes is a fat acceptance feed for a reason.

* That you have been blogging at your blog on a regular basis for at least 3 months about FA related issues.

* Blogs that express hostility to the Fat Acceptance

movement in general, that promote the idea of fat as unhealthy or negative, or promote weight loss as 'the answer', or refer to intended personal weight loss etc. will not be added to the fat feeds. Genuine self reflection is fine, blatant fat hate (yours or anyone else's) is not. Neither is bagging out other people you happen to think are too skinny, too fat, too ugly etc. We are not about condemning people because of their physical appearance.

\* Racist, sexist and ableist content will not be tolerated.

Big Liberty administers "The Fat Liberation Feed," which was a reaction to the strong liberal slant of the other feeds: "Originally started by fat libertarians, we recognized the need for a more politically balanced viewpoint of fat politics than allowed by the current status quo." This community is proving to be a space where fat individuals can go to find connection with like-minded individuals as well as information on fat acceptance, say Harding and Kirby.

Another entity that has been one of my saving graces and a boon to any scholar attempting fat positive work, the Fat Studies listserv, is designed to provide academicians a place to discuss fat positive issues. Marilyn Wann started the listserv in the summer of 2004 as a place for academicians studying fat positive topics to find support. As of the fall of 2011 the listserv had 627 members and many interesting conversations.

Fat positive entities are few and far between. Since I have been involved with this community I have watched the numbers grow significantly. Considering how many people are affected by the push to rid the world of fat people, however, the number is small. As more and more fat individuals find their voices, I expect the number and types of entities to grow.

## Fat vs. Overweight & Obese

THROUGHOUT THIS BOOK I USE THE WORD "FAT" RATHER than the medical terms "overweight" or "obese." The word "fat" has different meanings in different situations. For instance, when the medical community is discussing fat, they usually mean excess adipose tissue—actual fat cells. In the fat acceptance community, however, fat is more likely seen as a body size that is bigger than the socially acceptable size—a definition that is fluid and situated. NAAFA has actually described a fat individual as "an individual whose body weight exceeds that assigned to him or her by commonly accepted medical standards or who is commonly regarded as having excess weight." The fat acceptance movement prefers the word "fat" to words like "overweight" and "obese" since they consider the latter words to be artificially defined statements created by the medical community, Marilyn Wann writes in the foreword to *The Fat Studies Reader*. However, since the medical studies discussed in this book will all use these artificially defined terms rather than the more amorphous word "fat," when referring to such studies, I may use the terms "overweight" or "obese."

Another term that may appear in reference to body size is "societal ideal." When a fat individual uses this term, they usually mean someone who would not be considered "overweight" by the majority of individuals within the U.S. When speaking of medical studies, the ideal is usually called "normal." Controversy exists over terms such as "obese," "overweight," and "normal," controversy that has been exacerbated because the terms' definitions have changed with time and they are based on the Body Mass Index (BMI), which in itself is very controversial. For more information on definitions, see Chapter 2.

## *Health*

THROUGHOUT THIS BOOK I WILL BE DISCUSSING THE CONcept of "health," a term in which Americans put so very much stock. What is this health thing, anyway? The World Health Organization defines "health" as "a state of complete physical, mental and social well-being and not merely the absence of disease or infirmity." In the American Medical Association (AMA) general policy, the AMA defines health as "a state of physical and mental well-being." Few Americans could claim to be "healthy" given such definitions, especially considering the WHO's definition. Yet as a society we place a strong emphasis on striving for health—primarily physical health—above all else.

Many individuals in the fat acceptance movement resist defining health broadly and believe that individuals should determine what health means for themselves. "Health," Marilyn Wann asserts in the foreword to *The Fat Studies Reader*, "can be used to police body conformity and can be code for weight-related judgments that are socially, not scientifically driven;" she adds that the current idea of health reinforces "social control around [weight] and can be very damaging to well-being." Blogger Michelle, *The Fat Nutritionist*, discusses her own issues with the WHO definition of health, noting that it creates for a controlling culture:

> It's the silent assumption that anyone experiencing less than 'ideal' health is not only possibly to blame for their predicament, but that their lives are tainted, somehow broken, and possibly less meaningful than the lives of the 'healthy.'

> I propose that our definition of health should have less to do with how sick or well we are, and more to do with how we live inside and with our unique physical condition.

A person's state of health is what it is, and the thing to strive for is not less disease, or even longer life, but **the ability to inhabit, accept, and cope with what is....**

Are we banishing disease and improving quality of life, or are we blindly, almost compulsively, seeking to bring people in line with powerful, if latent, cultural ideals?

Michelle's ideas of health take the morality and control out of the concept. Kate Harding argues that health can be seen individually, that it should be defined "according to an individual's own body and its limitations." By changing their perceptions of the word "health," individuals can seek to resist societal control and find their own ideas of what "healthy" means.

That being the case, for this book, the word "health" will depend upon how it is used. At times I will be discussing American societal ideals about health. At these times the AMA's definition will be most appropriate. At other times I will be discussing how to strive for health as an individual. At those times, finding your own concept of health and what health means for you—physically, mentally, emotionally, socially, spiritually, etc.—will be most appropriate approach.

## Health At Every Size (HAES)

The HAES model is an alternative way of thinking about health that focuses on healthy behaviors rather than weight loss. One point to note, as mentioned by blog commenter Andrea on The Rotund, is that fat acceptance and the HAES approach, though compatible and like-minded, are not the same thing.

Linda Bacon, Ph.D. lists the following characteristics on the HAES Community website as the core principles of the HAES perspective:

• Accepting and respecting the natural diversity of body sizes and shapes.

- Eating in a flexible manner that values pleasure and honors internal cues of hunger, satiety, and appetite.

- Finding the joy in moving one's body and becoming more physically vital.

## Diet-medical-pharmaceutical-industrial complex (DMPI)

WHEN SPEAKING OF THE INDUSTRY THAT FINANCIALLY GAINS from the focus on weight loss, I use the term DMPI. Market-data Enterprises says this industry includes "diet soft drinks, artificial sweeteners, health clubs, commercial diet center chains, mail order and multi-level marketing diet plans, diet books and exercise videos, diet websites, diet food home delivery services, medically supervised programs (weight loss surgery, M.D.s, R.D,s, and nutritionist-based diet plans, hospital/clinic programs, Rx diet drugs, bariatrician plans), retail meal replacements and diet pills, low-calorie entrees and low-carb foods." According to Marketdata Enterprises, the weight loss industry made $60.9 BILLION in 2010, an increase from $58.6 billion in 2008.

# Rhetorical Success, Health Failure

AT THE WRITING OF THIS BOOK, THE "OBESITY EPIDEMIC" was proclaimed more than a decade ago. For all the focus on how bad fat is, we're not getting any slimmer, according to studies published in the *Journal of the American Medical Association* in January 2010. We have not seen a reduction in Type 2 diabetes, high blood pressure, or other problems supposedly associated with fat. What *has* happened? The American people are more than ever convinced that fat is bad, so prejudice against fat individuals has increased significantly. And our society has become terrified of fat.

If the "obesity epidemic" rhetoric was truly about health, ideas such as the HAES model would be gaining prominence as the focus on the "epidemic" increased. Instead, we have been seduced into believing that reduction in weight will solve our health problems, and that fat people are a problem to be solved.

Throughout this book I will show that the "obesity epidemic" is a campaign of manipulation started by those who wish to make a profit off of fear and self-hate—a project embraced by a society desperate for a prejudice perceived as justifiable. The dominant American society has made shallowness into an art form, lauding and moralizing actions that decades ago would have been seen as frivolous, self-mutilating attempts to control the uncontrollable. Many, many people are making a great deal of profit off of those attempts to control.

When it comes to rhetoric, to persuasion, the fight against the "obesity epidemic" is a rhetorical success, but an absolute health intervention failure.

# CHAPTER 2
## It's Not About Health, It's About Words

**I went to dinner with a good friend a while back. She seemed antsy and** restless while we were eating. Then excitedly she announced, "I'm on Weight Watchers!"

Wait—what?

She knows me well. She's heard me rail and rant about the failure of dieting. She's listened to me talk about fat acceptance. And yet she still had a thrill in her voice when she announced this to me. As I looked at her incredulously, she responded, "I know I only have a five percent chance, but this time I'm doing it for my health!"

As I stared at her in amazement, a light bulb went on in my head.

"But it's for my health" is often used as an almost mystical, magical talisman to ward off the gods of failed diets. There exists a belief that somehow, if people change their motivation, they'll lose weight. I believe this myth is behind the entire "obesity epidemic." We were starting to accept that diets don't work in the early 1990s—until, that is, someone came up with dieting for health. Then as a society we once again embraced dieting wholeheartedly; in fact, American society increased its fervor for weight loss. Now we MUST diet, because health is involved. And it would work this time, because it's "for my health."

When we consider the inception and focus on the "obesity epidemic," making fat about health instead of looks was an absolutely brilliant rhetorical move by the anti-fat industry. According to journalist Laura Fraser, in the early 1990s an anti-dieting movement started growing, emphasizing the fact that diets did not work. People appeared to be giving up on dieting for looks. American society started questioning the efficacy of trying to lose weight at all. This was the era of Susan Powter's very popular book *Stop the Insanity*, a book emphasizing the fact that diets did not work, though it maintained an emphasis on diet-like behaviors and weight loss. A 1992 NIH (National Institutes of Health) consensus panel also found that weight-loss dieting failed and was actually detrimental to the physical and psychological health of the individual, a statement that was later retracted and is no longer posted on the NIH consensus website. The movement against dieting continued to expand through the early 1990s.

The DMPI responded to this movement with a vengeance. Fraser says that researchers who had spoken out against dieting "found themselves once again underfunded." In another dazzling rhetorical move on the part of those making money from weight loss attempts, instead of arguing that weight-loss attempts worked—a proposition that had been repeatedly proven to fail—"obesity" researchers "raised the stakes by suggesting, with very sketchy substantiation, that obesity had become one of the nation's biggest health problems—a 'disease,'" says Fraser. Now fat became about health rather than aesthetics.

The American culture seemed to give a huge sigh of relief. The overall thinking appeared to be "dieting didn't work for our looks, but when we make it about health, it will work this time!"

Whereas beauty issues might not have appealed to everyone, making fat about health made fat a moral issue, giving it a much wider circle of influence, say both Paul Campos (law professor, newspaper columnist and author of *The Diet Myth*) and Eric Oliver (political scientist and author of *Fat Politics*).

Oliver notes that "we have created a disease out of a physical symptom that, in turn, we are unable to treat," and that "we are ascribing moral characteristics to what is largely a biological phenomenon." Campos calls the "obesity epidemic" a "moral panic," with fat individuals being relegated to the role of scapegoat.

This calling "overweight" and "obesity" a disease in and of itself creates a number of implications for the fat individual—implications that provide legitimacy to fat prejudice and discrimination and promote negative attitudes toward the fat person. Whereas the proponents of fat acceptance believe that fat is just normal human diversity, calling fat a disease seeks to force the fat individual into a narrow ideal of what is "normal." Since fat is seen as a disease, it must be eradicated at all costs, making extreme measures seem not so farfetched.

Moreover, the DMPI complex—this time working through the U.S. Surgeon General and other government entities—again made a smart move by calling the increase in rates of "overweight" and "obese" individuals in the U.S. an epidemic, a rhetorical move that has incredible implications for fat individuals and for attitudes about fat in this country.

To comprehend the rhetoric behind this move, we must first understand exactly how the jump in "obesity" and "overweight" came about, since the American people actually only weigh 6.5–11 pounds more, on average, than they did a generation ago, according to Campos, Saguy, Ernsberger, Oliver, and Gaesser. We are also about an inch taller. Since we have not had a huge jump in weight, how did this supposed growth spurt happen?

To start with, the DMPI complex lowered what it means to be "normal" versus "overweight" and "obese." The situation was exacerbated by the terms being based on the BMI—Body Mass Index—which in itself is very controversial. (See Eric Oliver's *Fat Politics* for an excellent examination of the controversy behind the BMI.) BMI is calculated by taking a person's weight in kilograms and dividing it by the square of his or her height in meters. The BMI formula was originally created by the Belgian astronomer Adolphe Quetelet, who was trying to detect criminals and deviants by their "physical abnormalities"—not just identifying, but problematizing those outside of the norm. Before 1998, the Centers for Disease Control considered men "overweight" at a BMI of 27.8 and women at a BMI of 27.3. In 1998 "underweight" was redefined as a BMI of 18.5 or lower, "normal weight" was redefined as a BMI of 18.5 to 24.9, "overweight" was redefined as a BMI of 25.0 to 29.9, and "obese" was redefined as a BMI of over 30.0. When the BMI criteria for the weight categories was redefined, 37 million people became "overweight" overnight without gaining any weight.

Because the BMI does not discriminate between muscle and fat, many of those in the "overweight" category are athletes, Campos asserts.

The change in weight classification came through a National Institutes for Health (NIH) Obesity Task Force that was pressured to conform to standards from the World Health Organization (WHO). The WHO standards came from a recommendation by the International Obesity Task Force, an organization funded primarily by two pharmaceutical companies who were marketing weight loss drugs, Hoffman-La Roche and Abbott Laboratories, according to Linda Bacon, a nutrition professor at City College of San Francisco and a leading advocate for the HAES approach.

Campos argues that the "obesity epidemic" is actually the result of statistical manipulation. By changing the definitions for "overweight" and "obesity," as noted above, an increase of a few pounds in the weight of the average American caused "a 61% increase in the obesity rate."

The change in definition gave impetus and momentum to the DMPI's propaganda being produced at the time. After the definition change, researchers and public health officials could honestly say the *rates* of "overweight" and "obesity" were growing alarmingly, not noting that *weight* actually was not. Campos explains that standards for children's weight have also changed as well:

> So we've gone practically overnight from a situation where 5% of America's children were defined as "overweight" according to an almost completely arbitrary definition, to one in which around 15% are now "obese" and more than 30% are "overweight," by even more radically arbitrary definitions—even though America's children weigh no more than they did ten years ago.

By changing the definitions of "overweight" and "obesity," the DMPI has created the appearance of huge weight increase when we have actually only experienced a slight enlarging of our population—a situation that has continued since the mid 19th century, says medical statistician T.J. Cole. Because of the redefinition of weight categories, the DMPI could now honestly claim a large jump in the incidence of people who fall into the "overweight" and "obese" categories.

On top of the redefinition, the category labels themselves are a rhetorical move creating negative implications for those who fall into the "overweight" and "obese" categories. The very definition of "normal," according to the *Merriam-Webster Dictionary*, implies conformity: "according with, constituting or not deviating from a norm, rule, or principle," or "conforming to a type, standard, or regular pattern." The word "normal" suggests that the majority would fit into this standard. In actuality, only 31.6 percent of the American population falls into the "normal" weight category, according to the National Institute of Diabetes and Digestive and Kidney Diseases (NIDDK).

Fat activist Marilyn Wann notes that such labels as "overweight" and "obese" medicalize human diversity and "are neither neutral nor benign." She also says that "overweight" implies "an extreme goal: instead of a bell curve distribution of human weights, it calls for a lone, towering, unlikely bar graph with everyone occupying the same (thin) weights."

As for the "obesity epidemic" itself, Oliver claims that William H. Dietz, M.D., Ph.D., the director of the CDC's Division for Nutrition and Physical Activity, started the idea of an epidemic. In fact, Oliver calls Dietz "patient zero" of the epidemic.

By using a PowerPoint slideshow to reveal the growing "problem," Dietz portrayed "obesity" as a disease slowly engulfing the U.S. "Simply by virtue of the visual presentation of the data," Oliver writes in *Fat Politics*, "the CDC maps could convince people that America's weight gain was, in fact, a real 'epidemic.'" The slides suggest some great scourge is slowly creeping over the country. Then, in 2001, a report—actually a high profile Call to Action from Surgeon General David Satcher—reinforced this idea by declaring that we were indeed experiencing an "obesity epidemic."

The word "epidemic...sounds an alarm bell" to the American people, Gordon R. Mitchell, Ph.D. and Kathleen M. McTigue, M.D., M.S., M.P.H. state, since it is a term "historically reserved for describing infectious disease outbreaks." The word has two potential meanings, they add, both with significant implications—the first a medical term implying an infectious disease that can be easily transmitted, causing quick and imminent death, and the second a rhetorical metaphor suggesting "the rising prevalence of excess body weight as a universal problem requiring collective response."

Using the term "epidemic" in referring to "obesity" makes fat about public health, not about an individual's wellbeing, and creates an atmosphere of urgency. This provides legitimacy for practicing fat prejudice as a culture, since people see "obesity" as a public health crisis that must be stopped.

Probably one of the most powerful implications of using the word "epidemic" comes in the idea that fat is spreading like a communicable disease. In other domination situations, privileged individuals, such as those who are white or male, do not have to worry about unwillingly becoming an individual who may experience oppression, such as African-Americans or women. Since, theoretically, anyone may gain weight, Americans have become obsessed with the fear of becoming fat, says Marilyn Wann.

Since we do gain weight as we age, since some pharmaceuticals cause weight gain, since depression can cause weight gain, since illnesses such as hypothyroidism or Cushing's syndrome can cause weight gain, there exists some truth to the belief that anyone can become fat at any time. This belief adds fuel to the thought that fat is contagious. One study by Nicholas A. Christakis, M.D., Ph.D. and James H. Fowler, Ph.D. even tried to suggest that fat is contagious through social networks, a conclusion refuted later by Ethan Cohen-Cole, Ph.D. and Jason M. Fletcher, Ph.D. Another study suggested that "obesity" is caused by a virus, though that has not been confirmed as of yet. In response to such worries as fat being a communicable disease, in 2006 an Australian healthcare conference hosted a symposium discussing the idea of outlawing "obesity."

Whoever came up with the idea of making dieting about health is simply brilliant. Now society can be prejudiced, but it's OK because it's about health. Now you are not shallow if you focus all your attention on dieting—you are righteous. And woe be to you who do not diet, for thou art sinning!

# *The Obesity Paradox*

THE TERM "OBESITY PARADOX" IS A RHETORICAL MOVE THAT creates significant implications for fat individuals. The results of studies that find fat is not problematic or may be even protective have been labeled as part of this paradox by the medical community because the results challenge the prevailing belief that fat in even small amounts is unhealthy.

The term "obesity paradox" first appeared in medical studies in a 2002 *Journal of the American College of Cardiology* article entitled "The Impact of Obesity on the Short-Term and Long-Term Outcomes After Percutaneous Coronary Intervention: the Obesity Paradox?" After that the term becomes more and more common, as the table reveals, with a significant increase in articles discussing the "obesity" paradox in 2008.

Whether or not a paradox exists in regard to "obesity" is no longer in question, as physician researchers Darren S. Schmidt and Abdulla K. Salahudeen state: "When the obesity-survival paradox was initially described 10 years ago, the argument was whether the phenomenon existed. Now, as evidence has continued to mount, the argument has shifted toward, 'What does the phenomenon mean?'"

| Year | PubMed |
|------|--------|
| 2001 | 0 |
| 2002 | 2 |
| 2003 | 1 |
| 2004 | 1 |
| 2005 | 7 |
| 2006 | 8 |
| 2007 | 10 |
| 2008 | 73 |

Occurrence of term
"obesity paradox"
on PubMed

There are also articles that can be classified as part of the "obesity paradox" but do not invoke the term. Flegal et al.'s 2005 *Journal of the American Medical Association* article entitled "Excess

Deaths Associated with Underweight, Overweight, and Obesity" is an excellent example of an article that said fat is not unhealthy and yet does not specifically refer to the "obesity paradox." When a study finds anything positive regarding fat, that study is considered part of the "obesity paradox."

The actual term "paradox" has a number of rhetorical implications. The *Oxford English Dictionary* defines paradox as "a statement or tenet contrary to received opinion or belief, esp. one that is difficult to believe." So by the very use of the word "paradox" we understand that studies that fall into this realm are considered divergent and difficult to accept. The term also implies an abnormality, a deviation from normalized behavior or belief. By using this term the medical community highlights the belief that fat is unhealthy in all situations, generalizing the health situation of all fat individuals. Studies that fall into the realm of the "obesity paradox" are contrary to the understood belief that fat is unhealthy. Once again, such language places the fat individual in the position of being abnormal and deviant.

The DMPI's rhetorical moves in creating the "obesity epidemic" have worked—perhaps beyond the originators' expectations. Fat has been demonized by the use of loaded words like "disease" and "epidemic," redefining terms to exaggerate population characteristics, and by using visuals to imply a spreading contagion. Examining the rhetoric behind the "obesity epidemic" shows us just how powerful rhetoric can be in manipulating public opinion.

People have been duped into thinking that fat is bad. And since they are trying to lose weight for their health, it will work this time.

# Chapter 3
## It's Not About Health, It's About Prejudice

Though the DMPI is behind the rhetoric that started the anti-fat movement, they did not have to push much to get the American public to believe fat is bad. Americans jumped on the idea that fat must be obliterated. Though we continually hear how the push to eliminate fat people is a move toward health, what we see in actuality is prejudice, stigma and oppression hard at work.

Can we really call the general American attitude toward fat individuals "prejudice"? The *Oxford English Dictionary* defines prejudice as a "[p]reconceived opinion not based on reason or actual experience; bias, partiality; (now) spec. unreasoned dislike, hostility, or antagonism towards, or discrimination against, a race, sex, or other class of people." Does American society as a whole have preconceived negative attitudes towards fat individuals based solely on their body size?

In their 2006 *Obesity* article "Confronting and Coping with Weight Stigma," psychologists Rebecca Puhl and Kelly Brownell summarized the perceptions of fat individuals:

Negative stereotypes include perceptions that obese people are mean, stupid, ugly, unhappy, less competent, sloppy, lazy, socially isolated, and lacking in self-discipline, motivations, and personal control.

We must also consider stigma, which is different from prejudice. Sociologist Erving Goffman defined stigma as "an attribute that is deeply discrediting." For the fat individual, according to psychologists Kelli E. Friedman, Jamile A. Ashmore and Katherine L. Applegate, stigmatized experiences include:

> Encountering physical barriers (e.g., not being able to find medical equipment in an appropriate size), people making unflattering assumptions toward the obese individual, being avoided, excluded, ignored because of weight, and receiving inappropriate comments from physicians.

Finally, do fat individuals experience oppression? *Merriam-Webster* defines oppression as "unjust or cruel exercise of authority or power." As I show in this book, fat individuals experience oppression in many areas of their lives.

Unfortunately, fat prejudice and oppression are both very easy to prove. Entire articles, even books, have been written detailing fat discrimination as a whole. Attorney Sondra Solovay's *Tipping the Scales of Justice* looks at the legal ramifications and solutions to fat bias, while J. Eric Oliver's *Fat Politics* looks at fat prejudice from a political science point of view. Each of these books is considered on the side of fat acceptance. Scholarly works with no connection to fat acceptance include Puhl and Brownell's articles "Bias, Discrimination, and Obesity" and "Confronting and Coping with Weight Stigma," and their 2005 edited collection, *Weight Bias.* Another is C.L. Maranto and A.F. Stenoien's "Weight Discrimination: A Multidisciplinary Analysis." A myriad individual studies establish prejudice in a number of situations. For the purposes of this book, I highlight only a few of the most interesting and relevant statistics.

Fatness can affect employment and wealth levels. Being fat can reduce a white female's net worth significantly—less so for black women and white men, and none for black men, says research scientist Jay L. Zagorsky in an article entitled "Health and Wealth: The Late-20th Century Obesity Epidemic in the U.S." In a 2001 article, Puhl and Brownell reported that fewer "obese" employees are being hired in high-level positions, while fewer "obese" individuals are being promoted. When given the same resume with different pictures of the same individual at different weights, college students ranked "obese" individuals as having "having less leadership potential, as less likely to succeed, and as less likely to be employed than normal-weight candidates," while assigning them lower starting salaries and considering them less qualified, a 2008 study by K.S. O'Brien, J.D. Latner, J. Halberstadt, J.A. Hunter, J. Anderson and P. Caputi found. Interestingly enough, another study found that individuals with a BMI over 35 experienced higher levels of perceived mistreatment when they were of higher socioeconomic status. Considering these statistics, we can see that being fat can affect individuals' opportunities for employment and wealth.

Researchers have found fat prejudice in medical situations as well. Doctors in Canada are moving fat patients to the bottom of the waiting list or refusing to treat them outright. "Obesity" experts—doctors treating "obesity," "obesity" researchers, and the like—often have a strong bias against fat individuals. Additionally, as much as 40 percent of physicians as a whole have negative attitudes toward "obese" individuals. Negative attitudes are so prevalent in the medical field, in fact, that fat individuals often hesitate to seek medical care.

"Only drug addiction, alcoholism, and mental illness aroused more negative feelings [in physicians] than obesity," argue A.N. Fabricatore, T.A. Wadden and G.D. Foster.

At least 50 percent of primary care physicians see "obese" individuals as noncompliant, while another study found primary care physicians tend see "obese" individuals as "awkward, unattractive, ugly, and noncompliant." A study of implicit attitudes of those who treat "obesity" found the physicians to have a strong anti-fat, pro-thin bias and a tendency to see "obese" patients as "lazy, stupid and worthless." Another study found that physicians recommended psychological counseling to "obese" patients significantly more often than to "normal" weight individuals, "suggesting a belief that those who are overweight must also be unhappy and unstable."

In short, a great deal of research suggests that fat prejudice is rampant in the medical field.

Perhaps the most disturbing consequences of fat prejudice include the experiences of fat children and adolescents. Children as young as preschool age already have anti-fat bias, and those with a caregiver who have anti-fat attitudes have higher levels of anti-fat bias. As many as 25 percent of adolescents report weight-based teasing throughout their adolescent years by their peers; 48 percent report teasing by both peers and family, with "obese" adolescents report a significantly higher incidence of teasing.

Though "obese" stereotyping is relatively consistent in all age groups, younger individuals experience more denigration in relation to attractiveness. "Overweight" adolescents who are teased experience a greater risk of disordered eating thoughts and behaviors, as well as psychological problems such as anxiety, low self-esteem, depression and anger. Most disturbing of all, prejudice towards fat children and teens appears to be growing, not diminishing. A recent study showed that fat children are six times more likely to be bullied than children who are not fat.

We cannot ignore the fact that fat prejudice is tied up with racism and classism. Fat is definitely associated with being poor and lower class. Fat individuals have a better chance of being poor, Paul Ernsberger, Ph.D. writes in *The Fat Studies Reader.*

Though we tend to believe as a society that poverty causes people to be fat, Ernsberger argues that fatness actually causes poverty—intelligent fat people are far more likely to end up living in poverty than are intelligent thin people. Ernsberger declares that "there is some evidence that poverty is fattening; there is much stronger evidence that fatness is impoverishing," a belief echoed by J. Fikkan and Esther Rothblum in their 2005 study.

If you think about it, arguing that being poor causes fat is another way for classist folks to once again say that poor people experience what they do by "choice," though in a roundabout way. However, if you say that being fat causes a person to be poor, that reveals society's prejudice and how it affects people. No wonder the focus is on how to save the poor from themselves rather than making society as a whole face the dominant prejudices—it is so much easier to blame the abused for the abuse. Added to the fact that being fat can reduce the socioeconomic status of an individual, poor individuals are more likely to sit at the high ends of their set points—the range of weight a body naturally maintains. (I will discuss set point in further detail later in this book.)

The idea that anyone can eat healthy food and exercise if they so desire does not take into account the situation for many individuals who live in poverty. Many individuals may not have a safe place to exercise, S.E. Parks, R.A. Housemann and R.C. Brownson note in a 2003 article comparing correlates of physical activity in urban and rural adults. Access to healthy foods is often limited in poverty stricken areas, a situation that is being called a "food desert." Additionally, many affordable foods provide high calories but low nutrition. However, although poverty does appear to exacerbate fatness, as noted above, fatness also appears to cause poverty. This can be a vicious downward cycle—a fat individual cannot find adequate employment, causing lower income, which causes less access to health care and healthy foods, which causes higher weight, which causes less access to adequate employment, leaving fat individuals more likely to experience poverty.

As we can see, scholarly work has established the incidence and prevalence of fat prejudice, stigma and oppression. A number of studies provide documented evidence of discrimination and bias towards fat individuals—discrimination and prejudice that almost doubled between 1996 and 2006 and now rivals race and age discrimination, according to T. Andreyeva, Puhl and Brownell. However, looking at the dominant rhetoric, our society does not believe that fat individuals deserve protection from discrimination since their situation is perceived as being self-induced and changeable. (For a closer examination of fat prejudice and how it works, see my upcoming book *Acceptable Prejudice? Fat and Social Justice in the U.S.*)

When the DMPI started talking about the "obesity epidemic," the American people grabbed hold of this prejudice and embraced it with self-congratulatory glee. Now prejudice was justified! These people could change, are unhealthy, and deserve to be treated poorly so they might make the effort to lose that weight! (All topics I will approach in this book.) For whatever reason—that humans have an innate desire to look down on others, that we like having scapegoats, that we want to feel superior to someone—America embraced fat hatred with a vengeance. This prejudice would be intolerable even if all these beliefs were true, but the fact that this prejudice is based on assumptions and misinformation makes it all the more horrifying.

# Chapter 4
## It's Not About Health, It's About Assumptions

The appeal to fairness and equity is of course logical. Most thoughtful people agree that discrimination just isn't okay and should not be tolerated. However, appeals to fairness have proven surprisingly uncompelling to most people when it comes to fat rights. The main reason appears to be that most people believe that fatness is a personal choice, a result of poor lifestyle habits, and that individuals deserve to hold responsibility for their choice. After all, the argument goes, if fat people want to escape discrimination, they should just lose weight—and thinner people should not have to absorb the costs of someone else's fatness, whether it's about sitting in a cramped seat or the taxes incurred from health care costs. In effect, this attitude often justifies more discrimination, with the belief that the unfair treatment may motivate people to lose weight.

Linda Bacon said the above in a talk at the 2009 NAAFA convention. She notes that the primary reason that fat prejudice is not acknowledged as oppression is this belief that fat is permanently changeable. Whether it be Jenny Craig's assertion that "we change lives," the Mayo Clinic's claim to provide "reliable information to achieve weight loss and maintain a healthy weight," or the Ad Council's campaign showing disembodied fat body parts as the reason for taking "small steps to get healthy," the American public is inundated with the message that weight loss is possible and necessary to obtain health—a message that supports the $60.9 billion weight loss industry. Fat individuals can often become temporarily thinner, leading the majority of persons—including fat individuals themselves—to believe that fat people can become slim with the application of enough willpower and effort.

Even the CDC claims that energy imbalance is the primary cause of "obesity:" "Overweight and obesity result from an energy imbalance. This involves eating too many calories and not getting enough physical activity." This statement reflects what could be seen as a commonsense understanding held by many people in the U.S. However, science does not support this equation.

As Glenn Gaesser, a professor and director of the Exercise and Wellness Program and the Healthy Lifestyles Research Center at Arizona State University, argued in an article entitled "Thinness and Weight Loss," little evidence exists that the "calories in equals calories out plus fat" equation has any merit. Additionally, medical science has not yet found an effective and safe way to keep weight off permanently for the majority of fat individuals, according to a number of sources including Gaesser, Bacon, and a meta study by psychologist Traci Mann and colleagues.

Weight gain can be caused by disease, medications or depression, yet many fat individuals are that way because of genetics, says research physician Albert Stunkard. Stunkard's twin studies show that about 70 percent of an individual's body size is determined by genetics.

*New York Times* science writer Gina Kolata, author of *Rethinking Thin: The New Science of Weight Loss—and the Myths and Realities of Dieting*, summarizes the issues with food and weight:

Some overweight people eat quickly, some slowly. Some binge, some do not. Some eat when they are stressed; some lose their appetites in those circumstances. And, in every case, thin people are just as likely as the obese to exhibit those behaviors. There is no behavior that is typical of the obese.

Study after study has shown that fat individuals eat no differently than their skinnier counterparts—some eat too much, some eat too little, and some eat a medium amount. Yet our society assumes that fat individuals just need to eat right and exercise—and that they must not be doing that—in order to be thin.

## Set Point Theory

SET POINT THEORY PROVIDES AN EXPLANATION FOR WHY most people cannot lose weight and keep it off. Set point theory suggests that our body has a particular range of weight that it is comfortable in—usually about 10 percent of a body's weight, "possibly 10 to 20 pounds," Linda Bacon argues. Bacon explains that a set point is:

- The weight you maintain when you listen and respond to your body's signals of hunger and fullness.

- The weight you maintain when you don't fixate on your weight or food habits.

- The weight you keep returning to between diets.

Most people lose and gain within this set point range. They may put on a little weight in the winter and lose it in the spring. Or get busy and drop a little weight. Or lose a little during an illness. Or gain a little during a stressful time. Movement within this range is normal. However, movement outside of that range is not, say researchers Richard Keesey and Terry Powley. In fact, the body seeks homeostasis. That means the body seeks to stay within this limited range of both weight and energy expenditure, Keesey argues. To move outside of this comfortable range something must go on—something must happen to the body.

The range appears to be set by a number of factors. The strongest factor seems to be genetic. A variety of adoption and twin studies have determined that about 75 percent of our weight is due to genetics. Albert Stunkard found that identical twins raised apart were almost as likely to resemble their twin's weight as those raised together, a result that was confirmed by H.H. Maes, M.C. Neale and L.J. Eaves. That other 25 percent is affected by a number of factors that can mess with set point, including disease. For instance, a great deal of evidence suggests diabetes causes individuals to get fat. Thyroid disease, Cushing's Disease, Polycystic Ovarian Syndrome (PCOS) and other diseases all cause weight gain. Medications can cause weight gain, or loss. Depression can also cause the body to gain or lose weight. Stress can cause gain or loss. And the kicker— DIETING can also mess with this homeostasis.

When something tries to change the weight of an individual, the body fights back. This is true of changes both up and down. A Vermont prisoner overfeeding study found that after the prisoners gained about 25 percent of their original body weight, their metabolism shifted so they could gain no more. Some were eating 10,000 calories a day just to maintain that gain. When they quit eating so much, their bodies returned to their original weight, for the most part.

When we try to lose weight, our bodies will let it happen for a time, but then they start fighting back. The body may adjust the metabolism to hold onto weight. It may start an almost voracious desire for high carbohydrate and high fat foods. Individual bodies may have different responses, but most will find the weight coming back on. And most bodies will increase the set point range, believing that they have experienced starvation and must protect against such danger again.

Now, a very small portion of the population may be able to reduce their weight and keep it off, if they are willing to spend a great deal of their time on maintenance—equivalent to a maintaining a part-time job, blogger DebraSY claims. She has found that maintaining weight loss requires an inordinate amount of dedication and focus. Such effort is seen as reasonable by American society as a whole. However, some fat people actually want to have a life, not just a weight maintenance regime.

My own personal opinion? For 40,000 years the primary threat to the majority of humans tended to be not getting enough to eat. In fact, this was true until the end of World War II in the United States, and is still true in many Third World countries (and for some in the West, as well) today. Since starvation was common, our bodies learned to hold onto weight at all costs. Anytime our bodies experience lack, they learn to be more efficient in holding weight—i.e., the body that experiences lack increases the set point. Children who experience famine have very efficient bodies—bodies designed to hold onto fat. People who experience starvation repeatedly will have bodies that get better and better at holding onto fat.

So how is the body supposed to tell between starvation and a diet? It can't. All the body knows is that the signals—signals of hunger or craving—it is sending are being ignored. And the only way it knows to respond is as if there is a famine. So it holds onto weight and creates a demand for high calorie foods. And so the diet fails for the majority of us.

With the incredible number of studies showing that dieting makes you fat, why are so many people still dieting, often at the suggestion of doctors? Deeleigh of *Big Fat Blog* noted three common responses to studies with such conclusions:

- Extreme dieting causes long term weight gain, but "sensible" diets or "lifestyle changes" don't.

- Some types of restricted eating cause long term weight gain, but others don't, i.e. "ur doing it wrong!"

- Weak-willed people gain more weight back after losing weight because they go nuts overeating after periods of restraint.

As pointed out before, whether you call it a diet or a life style change, for most people the weight still comes back on. For many people, even keeping up the maintenance behaviors will lead to weight regain.

The idea that anyone can lose weight and keep it off must completely ignore set point theory—a theory with a great deal of evidence backing it—in order to continue that belief.

## *The Sisyphean Bind*

THE BELIEF THAT WEIGHT IS CHANGEABLE CREATES AN IN-credible bind that fat individuals face when resisting oppression and the demand for weight loss. Fat individuals are expected to lose weight in order to overcome oppression. Society as a whole feeds individuals a message to be other than they are in order not to experience prejudice.

Fat individuals are told to lose weight to gain the rights and privileges afforded other individuals, but no effective solutions for losing weight have been found. This situation leaves fat individuals in an unachievable situation. They are expected to perform a task—a task proven to be unrealistic at best and impossible in many cases—in order to be treated like normal human beings.

This situation contributes to a form of prejudice that I characterize as the Sisyphean bind.

The concept of a double-bind is appropriate to a point in explaining fat prejudice, especially if we consider the definition of double-binds provided by Elizabeth Britt in her book *Conceiving Normalcy* —situations in which individuals cannot win; "simultaneous and contradictory experiences of control and constraint, success and failure, and order and discontinuity." Anthropologist Gregory Bateson and colleagues originally explained double-binds as conflicting messages which each negate the other. Fat individuals do experience mixed or double messages of this nature. For example, fat individuals are constantly told to exercise, yet individuals in the Fatosphere have reported being verbally or physically abused when they attempt to do so—such as the experience of Sarah the triathlete, at the beginning of this book.

I came across this phenomenon repeatedly in my research. For instance, on a thread on *Fatshionista* discussing biking, cjtremlett elucidates the experience of many fat individuals:

> Y'know, for all the blathering about exercise and weight loss and the stereotype of fat people being lazy, you'd think they might think we were doing something right when they see us fat folks exercising. Instead, they just seem to pile on the abuse. How the fuck are we supposed to get that exercise you keep telling us to get when we can't do it without being harassed?

Sirriamnis confirms this experience of ridicule in a conversation on exercise within Marianne Kirby's blog *The Rotund*:

> We're "supposed" to be getting exercise, presumably so we don't "offend" the masses, yet the gym is the place where a lot of people seem to feel it's OK to harass someone heavy, or at the very least make faces and flee as if our fat were contagious.

As these comments suggest, fat individuals can face a double-bind when exercising—they are told to exercise, yet experience bias and stigma when they attempt to do so.

Even when fat individuals go out of their way to comply with society's constraints, they are often thwarted. Take the example of Evan, a fat person attempting to fly Delta Airlines, as reported by *The Consumerist*. Trying not to impinge his body on others, he attempted to buy two seats. Delta informed him that they might not give him the seats together, or that they might take the second seat away.

So even when attempting to comply, fat individuals are often given conflicting messages. These conflicting messages—these double-binds—are a "rhetorical mechanism through which normalization does its work," says Britt. (See Chapter 8 for more information on normalization.)

Though fat individuals do experience double-binds, there is also a dimension to their experience that cannot be described by our understanding of double-bind.

Society inundates fat people with consistent messages to lose weight and that such weight loss is possible to maintain. We do not yet have a word for the bind in which these fat individuals find themselves. I choose to call the situation a Sisyphean bind—a demand that the individual succeed at a futile task, one that must be performed over and over again, before being considered worthy to receive what others are granted automatically. When I ran this concept past the scholars on the Fat Studies listserv, body liberation activist and author Marilyn Wann suggested a better term might be "Sisyphean imperative."

Going back to our example of Evan and Delta—even when Evan was trying to be a "good fat person" and not impinge himself on others, in an online comment to the *Consumerist* article Go Pug Yourself fed him the message that weight loss was desirable and possible:

> I'm tired of these people crying discrimination every time someone doesn't bend over backwards to accommodate

them. It's hard to lose weight but it can be done if you are willing to work hard and you have willpower.

Read the comments on almost any news story suggesting fat might not be an awful thing, and you will see comments like Go Pug Yourself's.

We can consider a task Sisyphean, says the *Oxford English Dictionary*, when it is "endless and ineffective." The term "Sisyphean" is based on the story of Sisyphus and his rock as told by Homer in *The Odyssey*. Zeus bound Sisyphus, because of the human's hubris, to the eternal task of rolling a rock up a hill only to watch it roll back down again. A great deal of recent research suggests that dieting usually creates more fat than it alleviates, as individuals tend to regain proportionately more fat tissue than they originally lost. Therefore, intentional weight loss particularly fits the concept of a Sisyphean bind because it sets an individual up for weight cycling, the endless losing and regaining of weight that results from most attempts at dieting. Fat individuals can usually lose weight—at times through almost Herculean effort—only to see the pounds come back even when they maintain their weight-loss-oriented behaviors.

In fact, many fat individuals blame dieting for weight gain, often associating dieting with eating disordered behavior. In a post on how dieting and self-acceptance are mutually exclusive, Kirby, writing as The Rotund, notes that "I'd tried the diet thing for 20 years! The only thing I'd gotten was fatter." In the same blog post, Arwen declares that each diet put "at least 5 and usually 10 [pounds] on me, often without me going off the diet." On the blog *Shapely Prose*, Hope asserts that "It is NOT a coincidence that when America become obsessed with dieting that more people started gaining weight...I personally have wrecked my metabolism through ED [eating disordered] behaviors." Also on *Shapely Prose*, Heather notes that she starved herself into her fattest weight ever. On the same post, Patricia comments that even while maintaining changed behaviors, and though her health was better, she regained the weight she had lost.

In responding to a post entitled "Reduced Fat" on *The Rotund*, deeleigh said that eating healthy and exercising still left her fat:

> Maybe I'm superimposing my experience onto others, but I know that for me, walking a couple of miles a day and working out 3-4 times a week, plus eating a very healthy diet and moderating portions (though not counting calories) results in me having a BMI that's still over 30.

Weight cycling, the common result of dieting, can be a frustrating experience for fat people, leaving them to experience the Sisyphean bind. So the very nature of dieting is a fruitless task that demands a great deal of energy with little—even negative—results for the vast majority of fat individuals. And yet society expects the fat individual to succeed at this futile task, rather than have society change to accommodate fat individuals.

## *Failed Bodies vs. Failed Diets*

WEIGHT LOSS ATTEMPTS, WHETHER THEY ARE CALLED A DIET or a lifestyle change, fail repeatedly. In a review of studies of the long-term outcomes of weight-loss diets, Traci Mann, a social psychologist, has found that weight-loss dieting not only does not lead to long-term weight loss, it may lead to weight gain—as many as 83 percent of individuals who attempt to lose weight will ultimately gain weight instead. A study in the April 2011 edition of the *American Journal of Clinical Nutrition* found that attempts at weight suppression predicted a future increase in weight. Voluntary weight loss in men has been consistently associated with weight gain. Even when maintaining diet and exercise, most dieting individuals gain the weight back. In fact, one study by A.J. Tomiyama and others found that low-calorie dieting is associated with higher levels of cortisol, which can lead to heart and blood pressure problems, as well as increased stress upon the body.

Traci Mann summed up the problems with dieting:

> the potential benefits of dieting on long-term weight outcomes are minimal, the potential benefits of dieting on long-term health outcomes are not clearly or consistently demonstrated, and the potential harms of weight cycling, although not definitively demonstrated, are a clear source of concern. The benefits of dieting are simply too small and the potential harms of dieting are too large for it to be recommended as a safe and effective treatment for obesity.

Paul Campos, a professor of law at the University of Colorado Law School and author of a book in which he treats the "obesity epidemic" as a court case *(The Diet Myth),* asserts that "the perverse paradox at the heart of the diet myth is that this myth creates exactly what it most fears and loathes"—dieting makes people fat.

More and more studies have shown that weight is mostly genetic and cannot be lowered in the long run. Linda Bacon argues that "weight gain is relatively easy, but the human body is just not designed to support weight loss." In her book *Losing It: America's Obsession with Weight and the Industry that Feeds on It,* journalist Laura Fraser notes that most medical researchers recognize that attempts at weight loss are "risky and short-lived," but the anti-fat industry—those who make money off of attempts at weight loss, such as pharmaceutical companies, bariatric surgeons, weight loss programs, authors of diet books, and producers of diet foods—asserts that doing something is better "than to allow people to remain fat"—not recognizing that most attempts at weight loss actually exacerbate the problem.

Such studies suggest that we have no evidence that healthy, permanent weight loss is possible, and attempts to lose weight are actually making people fatter. Yet when a diet inevitably fails, the fat body is blamed for the failure.

Bariatric or "weight loss" surgeries such as gastric bypass and Lap-Band® have been touted as the current solution to "obesity". These surgeries have been given such magical properties as curing diabetes. Starvation apparently produces the same effect on diabetes, a recent study by the British physician Roy Taylor found. Of course if you starve a person long enough, there will be no need for health care—they'll be DEAD! And when the individuals quit starving, the problem comes back.

Bariatric surgeries contain a high risk of complications as well as the risk of death. Around one percent of bariatric surgery patients die in the first month, with an overall five-year death rate of six percent that includes a significantly higher heart attack rate and a suicide rate four times higher than the general population.

We cannot just note that suicide rate and not consider the implications. For whatever reason bariatric surgery patients are four times more likely to kill themselves than the general population—that the surgery seemed to be the last chance for a fat individual to get thin, or that the person is left in a miserable state of health after the operation—the suicide rate is horrific. And for all those who committed suicide, more are living in despair.

For the much-praised Lap-Band®, though a study by Jacques Himpens and colleagues found zero mortality rate on the operating table, the long time mortality rate was 3.7 percent. Additionally, 39 percent of Lap-Band® patients had major complications; 22 percent had minor complications. In the end, over 50 percent had to have the band removed. Yet if you talk to those who experience such failures, their surgeons have tended to blame the fat person.

For example, in a heartfelt post on the Australian blog *A Fat Lot of Good*, Dee explains her own experience with weight loss surgery:

> My surgeon blames me for the weight gain. To the point where I refuse to go to him again. I will not be blamed for what is not my fault. I will not be called a liar by him just because I don't fit his profile of what someone with a band should be like. I am me and I am someone who remains fat even with a lap band. I know a lot of people are going to say that obviously I don't eat 'right', that it is obviously my 'fault' that I haven't lost weight. To that I call bullshit. Those people don't know me. They don't know what I deal with because I have this stupid device in me.

So even with weight loss surgery the fat individual's body is blamed for any failure.

When a diet fails—even when it fails 95 percent of the time—the fat body is usually accused of the failure. If a car, a high tech gadget or even a drug failed 95 percent of the time, we would blame the manufacturer. But when a diet fails—our society blames the fat body. Heidi at the blog *Hortus Delicarium* reflects on this idea by saying, "If any other industry sold a method (at a premium price) that failed over 90 percent of the time, they'd go out of business. Every single day, the diet industry and the media try to sell us the message that diets work and that we are the failures if we don't lose weight and keep it off."

jm commented on the blog *Shapely Prose* about just how hard it is to change that kind of thinking:

> My FA [fat acceptance] journey is still in its infancy, and I struggle a lot with the idea that I am "giving up" and am therefore, a total failure. I know logically that this is ridiculous, but I've been so programmed to equate weight loss with success—as many of you know, it's hard to change that kind of shit thinking overnight.

The same idea of a failed body can occur in other instances as well. Whether it's being sick—"I just recently found out I'm a type two diabetic and feel like a complete failure and just another unhealthy fat statistic" (A.) or not finding clothes that fit—"Because 'obviously' it was somehow my body's fault, rather than the clothing line designers'" (Unapologetically Fat)— fat individuals have to fight not to believe that their bodies have failed. When a chair broke, living400lbs reminded herself that the chair, which was rated for her weight, failed, rather than her body.

Lori considers how society would view other products that fail 95 percent of the time:

> the more I think about it, the more insane it seems. I honestly cannot think of any other human endeavor that over 95% of people who attempt it fail at. Can you imagine if we had literacy programs in schools that ended up with over 95% of students coming out illiterate, and then claiming that the problem was that those students just didn't try hard enough? If there was a birth control method that failed over 95% of the time, and we said the problem wasn't the method, but that people were just too stupid and lazy to use it correctly? If there were a language that 95% of people who tried to learn it failed miserably at, and we were told that the language itself was totally logical and easy to learn, but people were just too stupid to pick it up? It's just crazy that we see weight loss failure as a willpower issue, and we buy that women who have succeeded at pretty much everything they've ever attempted in their life, including some really freaking hard things, fail at weight loss because they are just too lazy and stupid to remember it's as simple as calories in, calories out.

Adding to this increase in a sense of failure regarding the body, fat individuals as a whole have been reported to experience phobic fears about everyday living including "feeling afraid to travel, feeling uneasy in crowds, feeling self-conscious with others, and having to avoid certain things or places because they are frightening," argue Friedman, Ashmore and Applegate.

We have seen such tendencies before when considering women's bodies, as S.G. Kohlstedt and H. Logino note: "Women even adopt this language themselves, viewing their own bodies as mechanisms that have failed them."

Fat individuals often experience a sense of failure at the fact that they cannot lose weight. I am not anti-dieting because I want people to remain fat. I am anti-dieting because it **does not work.** Believing that the diet is for health doesn't make the odds any better.

Remember: you did not fail—the diet did.

## *Extreme Measures: Expectations of Weight Loss*

FAT INDIVIDUALS OFTEN EXPRESS FRUSTRATION AT THE FUtility of weight loss attempts and the continual message that they just need to do more. Before becoming involved in fat acceptance, individuals I studied found weight loss support groups a source of these unrealistic expectations. On her *Body Love Wellness* blog, Golda Poretsky tells of a Weight Watchers® leader who suggested cough drops might be the reason she wasn't losing weight. In a blog post on *Shapely Prose,* Heather feels like she dieted herself into her highest weight ever.

At this point, I should point out that weight loss is possible for most people, though not all. For many fat individuals weight loss often involves starvation, extreme exercise and a complete focus of all life energies on losing weight—none of which leads to health or quality of life, nor does it usually lead to permanent weight loss. Yet my research suggests that fat individuals are expected to go to these extremes.

A common argument heard when debating the changeability of fat is "there were no fat people in concentration camps." Do a Google search on the phrase, and you will see that it's a common comment on fat positive or even fat neutral posts on the web. Such arguments lend credence to the belief often voiced in the Fatosphere that the emphasis on eradicating fat is not about health. The blogger Random Quorum dealt with such a comment from her husband in which he argued that some of the concentration camp survivors may actually have been healthy. Considering that a study by J.J. Sigal found those survivors "suffered from diseases of every organ system—the heart, the lungs, the stomach, and the skeletal system—from 50 to 800 percent more frequently than an extremely well selected comparison group," health is probably not the result of such extreme starvation.

This comment regarding concentration camps also implies that nothing short of torture and starvation should be used in the search for weight loss. Because fatness is seen as a choice rather than a physical attribute and is believed to be a source of ill health, society believes that degrading, shaming and generally rejecting fat individuals is suitable, since this lack of acceptance might motivate the individuals to lose weight. (See the popular TV show *The Biggest Loser*, for example). Fat people are being expected to take extreme measures such as starvation or mutilating healthy stomachs (bariatric surgery) in order to meet society's ideals, couched in terms of health for the fat individual. Though these arguments may seem farfetched to the average person, it has been suggested that such camps may be the solution to "obesity." Sondra Solovay points out an example in her book *Tipping the Scales of Justice*: Dr. Walker, the author of a nationally syndicated newspaper column, noted that the fat should be locked up in prison camps for their own good and for the good of society.

Just because people *can* lose weight with extreme measures

does not mean it is healthy, reasonable or a good idea.

Though such expectations seem fantastical and extreme, my research suggests that fat individuals experience such suggestions often. Many members of the Fatosphere reported situations in which such extreme measures were expected of them. For instance, many of the participants on the blog *Shapely Prose* voiced their aggravation in a post responding to a video editorial by George Lundberg, M.D., editor of *MedGenMed,* which argued that "obese" individuals should just stop eating: "All this while the simple answer is to stop eating; stop feeding the obese until they are no longer obese." When wondering how an individual is supposed to get work done while fasting, blog commenter Sniper said, "Oh, right. Being thin is more important than having a life." On the same post, Bree noted that Lundberg is encouraging "pro-ana behavior"— that is, pro-anorexic behavior. Auds had a very strong reaction to Lundberg's editorial:

> Fast?!? Holy shit. I love how quickly it goes from "hey, have some vegetables" to "the reason you're fat is because you eat food ever." Look everybody, I'm not saying you need to reenact a war crime that killed 1/3 of the people forced to endure it to be thin, just you know, stop eating like 50% of your meals. You're welcome! (THIS IS NOT A LICENSE TO EAT THREE MEALS A DAY.)

In a blog post considering the social source of fat-negative medical studies, Nuckingfutz noted that her weight loss support group also supported extreme measures to lose weight. When she complained that she was not losing weight while walking 30-plus miles a week, they suggested she do more:

> They told me I had to do MORE, that 6 miles a day "obviously wasn't good enough." WTF? Fuck that shit… I had more important things to do (like cleaning the house, taking care of the children, doing the laundry, cooking) than to spend my ENTIRE DAY doing noth-

ing but exercise, just in the quest to become thin.

In a blog post on fat health care, Zan illustrates that even pharmaceutical drugs could be extreme measures, by saying "And Alli? Come on. Crapping your pants for a few extra pounds? Uh, no."

My research participants found that they were often expected to take extreme measures—often unhealthy ones—in order to lose weight. Professional dancer Ragen Chastain explained her viewpoint before practicing the HAES approach:

> I had bought into the diet industry's marketing that doing unhealthy things to get thin would lead to a body that was healthy, and that I couldn't be healthy until I was thin. Looking back it doesn't make any sense to me but at the time somehow it did.

Once again, we find evidence that the fight against "obesity" has nothing to do with health, since fat individuals are expected to practice extreme behavior in order to get thin.

# *Lack of Education*

THE DOMINANT MESSAGES OFTEN PROCLAIM THAT A LARGE part of the "obesity" problem is lack of education. We can see an example of this on the page discussing "obesity" on the National Heart, Lung, and Blood Institute (NHLBI) website:

> The National Heart, Lung, and Blood Institute (NHLBI) of the National Institutes of Health launched the Obesity Education Initiative (OEI) in January 1991. The overall purpose of the initiative is to help reduce the prevalence of overweight, obesity, and physical inactivity in order to lower the risk, and overall morbidity and mortality, from coronary heart disease (CHD). In addition, reducing the prevalence of overweight/obesity will help to prevent or improve other diseases and conditions such as Type 2

diabetes and sleep apnea.

Another example, First Lady Michelle Obama's campaign to reduce childhood "obesity," includes information on nutrition and exercise. Fat acceptance advocates do not argue that nutritional education is not a good idea—rather, they argue that nutritional education will not make anyone thin. By the time they are adults, fat individuals tend to be more aware of calorie-counts, nutritional value and fat content in foods than normal weight individuals. Eric Oliver, in fact, calls the nutrition education approach "a paternalistic condescension" that contains elements of racism and classism toward individuals who "are too ignorant to know that they should be thin." The fat acceptance movement does not argue against nutritional education, but against the idea that such education will reduce the levels of "obesity" in this country.

# Eating Disorders & Disordered Eating

IMPLICITLY OR EXPLICITLY, THE OVERALL BELIEF IS THAT ALL fat individuals experience disordered eating. In fact, the National Eating Disorders Association (NEDA) lists "overweight and obesities" along with disorders like anorexia and bulimia. Many people believe that fat individuals are fat because of issues with mental health. As reported in Gina Kolata's book *Rethinking Thin*, physician-researcher Albert (Mickey) Stunkard explored the idea that fatness was caused by a variety of emotional or psychological issues. What he found, however, was that fat individuals did not differ from their thinner counterparts in the severity or type of mental illness. He found no mental illness suffered only by "obese" individuals. "There is no psychological problem that is unique to fat people," Kolata reiterates.

Fat individuals are often believed to have Binge Eating Disorder (BED). Though not currently in the current version of the psychiatric diagnosis guide the *Diagnostic and Statistical Manual of Mental Disorders, Fourth Edition (DSM-IV)*, BED has been proposed for the *DSM-V*. The proposed definition would include:

A. Recurrent episodes of binge eating.

B. The binge-eating episodes are associated with three (or more) of the following:

1. Eating much more rapidly than normal

2. Eating until feeling uncomfortably full

3. Eating large amounts of food when not feeling physically hungry

4. Eating alone because of feeling embarrassed by how much one is eating

5. Feeling disgusted with oneself, depressed, or very guilty afterwards

C. Marked distress regarding binge eating is present.

D. The binge eating occurs, on average, at least once a week for three months.

E. The binge eating is not associated with the recurrent use of inappropriate compensatory behavior (for example, purging) and does not occur exclusively during the course Anorexia Nervosa, Bulimia Nervosa, or Avoidant/Restrictive Food Intake Disorder.

No doubt, some fat individuals do experience binge eating—about eight percent, argues Jon Robison, Ph.D., a professor of holistic health care at Western Michigan University. Interestingly, many will trace their binge eating back to restriction, Robinson says on the Association for Size Diversity & Health's *Health At Every Size* blog. After completing a literature review of studies that looked at BED, Robinson notes his frustration at the circular reasoning of the researchers (emphasis in the original):

> In the same articles identifying **deprivation** as the **main cause** of **BED**, the next paragraph or page would invariably go on to discuss how **dieting** and **restriction** might be a **good treatment** for **BED**! What? I had to go back a number of times to make sure I was reading this properly—and I was; everything from moderate dietary restriction to low fat, low density regimens to Very Low Calorie Diets were being recommended! No, you didn't just warp back into the previous millennium—I said Very Low Calorie Diets (VLCDs).

Robison argues that to find solutions for BED there is "a tremendous amount of paradigm-busting work to be done in transitioning from a weight-centered to a health-centered paradigm," and that the HAES approach may well be a successful intervention.

So only a small portion of fat individuals experience binge eating, yet our society tends to see fat individuals as binge or compulsive eaters. Meowser put it quite appropriately in a comment on the blog post "The Elephant (So to Speak) in the Room" on *Shapely Prose*:

> Fat acceptance doesn't say, "There's no such thing as a person who eats herself fat." Fat acceptance *does* say, "You can't *assume* all fat people have eaten themselves fat, and you can't tell who has and who hasn't just by looking, and *it's a private and personal fricking issue anyway, not some horrible morality violation, so butt the hell out.*"

When the fat individual is seen as disordered, "obesity" itself is pathologized. For example, NEDA listing "obesity" as an eating disorder shows that the organization considers the fat body itself disordered, because of the assumption that all fat people must be fat because they eat too much.

For the sake of those suffering from all eating disorders, we need to separate weight from behavior and focus only on the behavior. For those who truly do have the eating disorder of binge eating, one of the most frustrating elements of this focus on eliminating fat is that the current popular solution is a diet or some other form of restricted eating—a situation that fails continually, often making the disorder worse, with the failure commonly blamed on the sufferer of the eating disorder, like any other failed dieter.

Psychotherapists Jane Hirschmann and Carol Munter say that many binge eaters who quit dieting will quit bingeing. Stunkard also found that many individuals who suffer from BED are not fat, and their symptoms are often overlooked because of it. Our current solution for binge eating disorder is actually the *cause* of the disorder, and isn't helping the very people who need it!

Additionally, the diagnosis of anorexia needs to be separated from weight. A few of my research participants report having all of the symptoms of anorexia except for the required underweight BMI. For instance, Rachel at *The F-Word* tells in her story how being anorexic made her "normal" size, not underweight. The current *DSM-IV* says that to be anorexic an individual must experience "weight loss leading to maintenance of body weight less than 85 percent of that expected; or failure to make expected weight gain during period of growth, leading to body weight less than 85 percent of that expected." Therefore, a fat individual cannot be labeled anorexic and must fall into the EDNOS (Eating Disorder Not Otherwise Specified) category. Though it looks like the specific number will be taken out in the *DSM-V*, the revised definition still includes excessively low body weight. Therefore, fat individuals who suffer from all the other symptoms of anorexia will not be able to get the medical and psychological help they need because they are not in the "correct" weight zone. In fact, many suggestions for weight loss are often the same tricks anorexics use to keep weight off. Fat individuals are often actually encouraged to adopt anorexic behavior.

This belief that all fat individuals experience disordered eating is leading our medical community to approach fat in an ineffective and faulty manner.

At this time there appears to be a move in the dominant rhetoric to see the fat person as sick, overeating because of a brain disorder rather than morally lacking in willpower. For example, J.C. Lumeng, the author of a study on "obese" children and bullying, explains, "Obesity is really complex. It's not all about willpower. It's a brain-based disorder, and I hope that message becomes clearer."

This makes the fat person into a victim, rather than just a variation of human—once again emphasizing the otherness and the believed disordered nature of the fat individual. And the assumption is still that the fat individual is fat purely because of eating too much.

Yet we cannot ignore the effect that the focus on eliminating fat has produced in the rise of eating disorders and disordered eating. Not only are incidences of anorexia and bulimia increasing at an alarming rate in teenage girls, but they are increasing in women and men of all ages, according to the Academy for Eating Disorders (AED). Eating disorders are also showing up in younger and younger children. The Healthcare Cost and Utilization Project (HCUP) says that hospital stays to treat eating disorders increased 119 percent from 1999 to 2006 in children under 12. In addition, up to 30 percent of girls are estimated to have anorexic or bulimic eating habits, says a study by Bonnie Spear (though the AED only claims 10 percent).

According to Spear, we can connect dieting behaviors to an

increase in eating disorders all around. Dieting is only exacerbating the problem. One of the primary precursors to the prevalence of eating disorders is the incidence of dieting. As Fraser writes, "[A]lthough every diet doesn't lead to an eating disorder, *almost every eating disorder begins with a diet.*" (Emphasis in the original).

And now they are putting infants on diets, thanks to a new study by the Institute of Medicine suggesting that to prevent fat adults we must not have fat children—to prevent fat children, we need to reign in those babies. Given the experience of fat adults I have interviewed, these children will probably become fatter because of these interventions, and will struggle with weight issues, food issues and disordered eating their entire life.

In dealing with eating disorders, the one thing fat acceptance proponents discourage is weight-loss-focused dieting:

> However, focusing on weight is in my opinion couterproductive in the treatment of ANY eating disorder (yes, including binge eating and compulsive overeating). I cannot speak for you, but dieting, making rather unrealistic weight loss plans, and feeling disgusted by my body and my eating behavior are all just as much part of my ED as binge eating is.
>
> queendom *commenting on Kate Harding's post*
> "The Fantasy of Being Thin" *on* Shapely Prose

My research suggests that fat acceptance and the HAES approach can assist sufferers of eating disorders. Blog commenter Mshell67 came to *Shapely Prose* trying to figure out how a binge eater fit into fat acceptance:

> I'm feeling awful right now because I feel conflicted about my eating. I definitely have an eating disorder (I woke up at 3:00 am and ate frosting out of the can) and other such shit. So yesterday I felt like crap about myself and ate myself into a binge-o-rama. So, my question is,

would it be awful if I went to a counselor to discuss my binge eating issues in order to tame them a bit? What happens if I happen to lose weight? Am I a failure as a fat activist? Where do I fit in in this framework?

In response, Kirby, writing as The Rotund, argued that mshell67 should go see a counselor, that suffering from an eating disorder and being a fat activist was not mutually exclusive. "Breaking away from disordered eating," she said, "is not the same as controlling and limiting your diet for the express purpose of losing weight." Fillyjonk responded by noting that fat acceptance should be supporting those with eating disorders:

> I think you should expect—nay, demand!—that the fat acceptance movement buoy you up in your mission to eat in a way that is not harmful to you. Honestly, the fight against diets and the fight against binge eating or compulsive eating are two sides of the same coin: both are about healing our relationship with food, which is so drastically fucked up so early in life, and both are served by embracing HAES and unhitching health from weight.

Btsu thought counseling would be a great idea as long as it was a fat-neutral environment. Considering these conversations, members of the Fatosphere see the HAES approach as a possible solution to eating disorders. Whatever the solution, our current attitudes on fat and food are only making matters worse.

# *I Don't Want to Hear It*

YOU WOULD THINK THAT FAT INDIVIDUALS WOULD BREATHE A sigh of relief at hearing that fat isn't changeable. Experts often tout this belief when arguing against fat acceptance. For instance, in an online article touting the dangers of fat, Michael Fumento, a senior fellow at the Hudson Institute in Washington, noted in an attack on the anti-dieting movement that "say one thing for the fatlash activists and their journalist mouthpieces, they're singing a sweet Siren song that many fat people are dying to hear." In contrast, I have had people sneer or laugh at my work, but when someone gets upset at me, even furious, they are almost always very fat.

In my experience, most fat people desperately want to be thinner and will try anything and everything to get that way. In the results of a study on fat individuals' attitudes towards their own fat, psychologist Marlene Schwartz and colleagues at Yale University provide a list of disturbing trade-offs individuals would make in order to not be fat:

> Forty-six percent of respondents reported that they would be willing to give up at least one year of life rather than be obese, and 15% reported that they would be willing to give up 10 years or more of their life. In addition, 30% of respondents reported that they would rather be divorced than obese, 25% reported that they would rather be unable to have children than be obese, 15% reported that they would rather be severely depressed, and 14% reported that they would rather be alcoholic.

These are not people who are looking for an excuse to stay fat. By the time individuals have made it to fat acceptance, most have tried *beaucoup* diet products and weight loss schemes. Many have had weight loss surgery and other extreme measures, only to have that solution fail like all the others.

Of course most fat individuals want to be slimmer. When I tell them they have very little chance of ever being slim, I am telling them that, with our society as it is, they will always be socially unacceptable.

For larger individuals—what the Fatosphere jokingly refers to as "deathfat" as a play on the term "morbidly obese"—leaving their homes opens them to criticism and ridicule. At best, they'll likely be ignored. At worst, they may be ridiculed, mocked, given "concerned" advice, or out and out attacked. When I tell someone they have no hope of being thinner, I tell them they have no hope of this changing, unless they are willing to fight in order to change society—a much bigger job than a diet. No wonder people are willing to mutilate their bodies and risk death in order to be thinner. That is, most fat individuals would do anything to be socially acceptable.

In sum, fat individuals are expected to change what for many is unchangeable rather than having society change its prejudice. They are expected to go to extreme measures to lose their fat, whether or not those measures are healthy. This leads the fat person to experience double-binds, the Sisyphean bind, and a sense of failure. Society's demand that a fat individual become thin—seen as an attempt to make everyone the same—is actually just a way to make the fat individual into "the Other."

Again and again, we see the failure of weight loss attempts. This failure comes from one simple assumption that our society has taken hold of and refuses to consider, even though huge amounts of evidence exist to refute it and little (possibly none) exists to support it—that fat people are fat because they eat too much and exercise too little. Cultural rhetorics reinforce the belief that fat is changeable and possible, creating an unwinnable situation for the fat individual. This belief that fat is mutable, changeable, is the basis for the oppression fat individuals face daily. This belief makes fat a socially acceptable prejudice.

# Chapter 5
# It's Not About Health, It's About Correlations

**[The doctor said] "PCOS [Polycystic Ovary Syndrome] isn't a** real disease, it's been made up by fat women." I said, "I just had a biopsy about eight months ago," and she said, "we can't trust the results of those tests. If they told you you have PCOS they are quacks and are not interpreting the results correctly. You need to do what I say."
*Susanne on the blog* First Do No Harm

When I told her that I hadn't had a period in three months and that there was no possible way I could be pregnant, she immediately came back with "It's because you're overweight." She then told me to "shut my mouth once in a while" and to lay off the junk food.
*Emily on* First Do No Harm

These quotes reveal one of the greatest challenges for fat individuals—the medical community and health-related rhetorics. As suggested by my research into the experience of fat individuals as well as into medical studies, science and pseudoscience are being used to justify fat prejudice. In American society, we continually hear how "obesity" is killing us, how our children will be the first to die before their parents because of "obesity," and how we must strive to be thinner at all costs.

66

These claims give credence and power to attempts at eradicating fat.

The medical establishment is a very powerful entity within American society. Medicine is a rhetorical system, as rhetorician Judy Segal noted—"rhetorical as a system of norms and values operating discursively." In other words, medicine is based in persuasion, with established standards that function through subtext or overt communication. Given that "medicine is a powerful scientific and social institution," as medical rhetorician Ellen Barton says, resisting such an institution can be a daunting task. Yet that is a task that fat individuals face continually.

In order to understand exactly how medical rhetoric has been used to legitimize fat prejudice, in the following section I look more closely at the rhetoric—the communication—surrounding the idea that fat in and of itself is unhealthy, as well as other factors affecting fat individuals' health.

## Fat Not Unhealthy in Itself

BY LOOKING AT MEDICAL RHETORIC AS WELL AS CULTURAL responses to such arguments, we can see how fat prejudice has come to be legitimized and even lauded in today's culture. A quick search of the PubMed (NCBI) database reveals just how focused the medical research establishment has become on "obesity." From 1995 to 1998, 4,979 articles were published that had "obesity" as a primary topic; from 2006 to 2009, the same number of years, 19,942 articles were published on the topic of "obesity."

Though cultural rhetorics most often portray fat as overwhelmingly unhealthy, there exists quite a bit of controversy in the medical community regarding that belief. The current hype over "obesity" in the U.S. is directly connected to our ideas of health and what that means. In the forward to *The Fat Studies*

*Reader*, Marilynn Wann says that these ideas behind health are "socially, not scientifically, driven" and can be used to enforce conformity.

Fat individuals often face pressure to attempt weight loss for the sake of their health because our society has an intrinsic belief that fat is unhealthy, a belief that has been inflated by the "obesity epidemic." For example, the CDC lists the medical consequences of fat as:

• Coronary heart disease

• Type 2 diabetes

• Cancers (endometrial, breast, and colon)

• Hypertension (high blood pressure)

• Dyslipidemia (for example, high total cholesterol or high levels of triglycerides)

• Stroke

• Liver and Gallbladder disease

• Sleep apnea and respiratory problems

• Osteoarthritis (a degeneration of cartilage and its underlying bone within a joint)

• Gynecological problems (abnormal menses, infertility).

In reality, the medical establishment tends to be conflicted regarding whether or not fat actually causes these problems. Studies exist concluding that diabetes is caused by fat—yet studies also exist arguing that diabetes causes fat. Studies exist that argue fat is a primary cause of heart disease, yet a 2010 study by G.D. Batty, G. Der, M. Benzeval and I.J. Deary argues that fat is not one of the five top leading causes of heart disease. A study suggests that gallbladder problems can even be caused by weight loss. Some studies show the protective quality of fat in patients with heart problems and those on kidney dialysis. Though the dominant belief is that fat is unhealthy, a great deal of argument on that fact actually exists in the medical community.

In addition to the studies showing the out-and-out positive aspects of fat, we also have studies that fall into the previously mentioned "obesity paradox." In these studies we can find that fat provides many positive aspects to health:

- "Obesity" actually protects a patient post-operatively. "Overweight" and "obese" individuals had a decreased risk of death in post-surgical ICU.

- "Obese" patients with type 2 diabetes have lower mortality rates—they live longer. Higher mortality was associated with weight loss in type 2 diabetic patients, while weight gain did not change mortality rates.

- "Obese" individuals with type 2 diabetes had lower incidences of amputation as well as better post-operative outcomes after amputation.

- Weight gain actually helped those with cardiovascular disease.

- "Obesity" protected against respiratory failure in post-op patients.

- COPD patients with a higher BMI have a better long-term survival rate.

- A number of recent studies show that fat individuals have better outcomes after a stroke.

The list goes on. These studies show yet more proof that fat in itself is not unhealthy.

Many studies exist—and more are being produced—that

question the harmful nature of fat in itself. For instance, the prevailing rhetoric says that fat individuals die earlier than "normal" weight individuals. However, in a CDC study published in the *Journal of the American Medical Association* in 2005, Flegal, Graubard, Williamson, and Gail actually found that "overweight" (medically defined as a BMI of 25.0 to 29.9) individuals live longer than "underweight" (medically defined as a BMI of 18.5 or lower) or "normal" weight (medically defined as a BMI of 18.5 to 24.9) individuals. (For a more in-depth discussion of weight terminology, see Chapter 1.) Studies in Japan and Canada came to much the same conclusion as Flegal's team. In fact, many athletes fall into the "overweight" and even "obese" categories, argues Paul Campos. Yet Americans continue to believe that excess weight causes health problems.

For those diseases and conditions that truly can be associated with higher weights, fat acceptance proponents argue that these situations are often examples of correlation, not causation. For example, one argument from the dominant rhetoric is that "obesity" causes diabetes. However, a number of studies show the opposite, such as the previously mentioned studies showing that diabetes causes "obesity." Causation is very hard to determine. Since so many fat people diet and regain their lost weight, it may be weight cycling (repeated episodes of weight loss and regain) that is causing problems. Since fat individuals face prejudice and oppression daily, it may be the stress of stigma that is causing these conditions.

It may be that fat is a symptom of medical issues, rather than a cause. Since thin people get every disease associated with fat, fat is not likely the cause of any disease.

# *Thin Does Not Mean Healthy*

ONE OF THE GREATEST DANGERS OF THE FIGHT AGAINST "obesity" is the underlying assumption that thin people are healthy simply because they are thin. Study after study has shown this is not the case. Considering Flegal's research, we can see that underweight individuals actually have a younger mortality than "overweight" individuals and about the same mortality as "obese" individuals.

People who fall into the "underweight" and "normal weight" categories get sick and die—sometimes in preventable ways. Yet the assumption that fat individuals must be unhealthy gets turned around to where thinner individuals believe they are healthy simply because of their weight. By assuming that thin individuals are healthy just because they are thin, we do them a great disservice, Linda Bacon states.

"By putting an emphasis on weight," Bacon writes in her book *Health At Every Size*, "we also limit our ability to support thin people in adopting healthy behaviors."

Bacon argues that by focusing on weight loss, thin individuals—especially children—who have bad health habits get ignored. Additionally, Bacon notes, pushing for weight loss leads thin individuals to fear fat and may lead to eating disorders.

So our push to eliminate fat is just as damaging to thin individuals as it is to fat individuals. For the sake of everyone, we need to switch our focus to healthy habits instead of a narrow weight margin.

## *Effects of Dieting & Stress*

EXAMINING THE DATA PROVIDED BY MEDICAL STUDIES REveals a very weak connection between health and weight, yet a strong connection between health and behavior. Interestingly, when studies control for factors such as weight cycling, fitness, and activity, researchers tend to find little or no connection between body size and poor health indicators, Campos, Saguy, Ernsberger, Oliver, and Gaesser found in their 2006 *International Journal of Epidemiology* article. Weight cycling, a common result of dieting, may actually cause higher mortality rates, Traci Mann and colleagues argue.

In his book *Big Fat Lies*, exercise physiologist Glenn Gaesser argues that because of the nature of weight loss attempts—usually eating more nutritious food and exercising—no evidence exists that intentional weight loss *in itself* leads to a healthier body. Though the constant message provided by society says that the only way to improve health in "overweight" individuals is to lose weight, studies suggest that many health indicators can be improved by exercise and changes in eating habits that do not involve calorie restriction—ideas that are incorporated in the HAES philosophy.

More and more studies are showing that dieting for weight loss creates health problems in itself. A study has linked dieting to gallbladder issues. Protein-rich diets—diets like the Atkins diet—can cause the formation of kidney stones. As Deeleigh said on *Big Fat Blog*, "That's why a higher incidence of kidney stones is associated with "obesity;" because fat people are more likely to diet and have weight loss surgery." Bacon notes that weight cycling is "strongly associated with increased risk for diabetes, hypertension, and cardiovascular diseases, independent of body weight," arguing that dieting may actually be *causing* the health issues it supposedly prevents.

More research needs to be done on the effects of cortisol, especially in relation to diabetes. We know there is a connection between cortisol and diabetes, because increased cortisol levels increase blood sugar levels. We also know that continued stress will increase cortisol levels and that fat prejudice causes stress. Low calorie dieting also increases cortisol levels. So stress and dieting can increase a body's cortisol level, which in turn increases an individual's chance of having diabetes.

So, then, this demand that we lose weight may actually be causing the problems that weight loss is supposed to prevent! Peter Muennig, M.D., a medical researcher at Columbia University, actually argues this point in his *BioMed Central Public Health* article "The Body Politic: the Relationship Between Stigma and Obesity-Associated Disease."

Could the increase in fat prejudice actually be blamed for fat people experiencing higher levels of diabetes? Now THAT would be an interesting study. I suspect we would find a correlation between an increase in fat stigma and an increase in the prevalence of diabetes—although the correlation alone, of course, would not prove causation.

Another area where fat individuals may experience threat falls into what blogger, dancer and fat activist Ragen Chastain calls "The Vague Future Health Threat (VFHT)." Fat individuals who are healthy, and plenty of them do exist, are often threatened with future ills—diabetes, heart problems, etc. We do know that the concept of self-fulfilling prophecy has some merit even in health realms, a fact proven by the nocebo and placebo effects, if nothing else. What if these threats of future health ills actually lead to those future health ills? What if the stress of thinking they will get diabetes or heart disease leads individuals to a higher incidence of these diseases?

Worrying about what ails are to come may actually be doing much more harm than fat ever did. Besides, as Chastain says, "Everyone is going to die. There is a 100 percent chance."

Studies suggest that many of the ills—both physical and psychological—that fat people do experience may well be related to the stigma of being fat rather than the fat itself. For instance, physicians are likely to spend less time with fat patients, and are less likely to order appropriate tests for fat patients, while ordering a number of unneeded tests.

Considering that thin people who live with fat people have an increased risk of illness and death, as a study by J.T. Gronniger found, genetics and environmental factors are more likely the cause than is fat itself, Paul Ernsberger, Ph.D. argues. In fact, diseases linked to fat, such as diabetes and heart disease, are also linked to poverty and minority status. Since minorities and poor individuals are more likely to be fat, says Ernsberger, the correlations might point to causation there as well.

Muennig has found that the stress of experiencing weight-related stigma actually increases mortality, as does the desire to lose weight:

> Women who say they feel they are too heavy suffer more mental and physical illness than women who say they feel fine about their size—no matter what they weigh... Stigma and prejudice are intensely stressful. Over time, such chronic stress can lead to high blood pressure and diabetes.

We cannot ignore the effects of stress on the fat body—stress that has significantly increased since the advent of fighting the supposed "obesity epidemic." For larger individuals, stress is a very natural part of life. Individuals on the Fatosphere have reported everything from verbal abuse to out-and-out physical attacks because of their fatness. A truly fat individual can experience everything from being ignored to being physically and verbally assaulted when leaving home. This level of stress cannot help but hurt the physical health of the individual. Add to that the lack of self-esteem and feelings of failure created by dieting, as Linda Bacon found, and you get quite a formula for bad health:

> The health at every size group also demonstrated a parallel improvement in self-esteem, and 100% of participants reported that their involvement in the program helped them feel better about themselves (compared with 47 percent of the diet group). The diet group, on the other hand, demonstrated initial improvement followed by a significant worsening of self-esteem at follow-up. This damage to self-esteem was reinforced in other of the self-evaluation questions. For example, 53 percent of participants in the diet group expressed feelings of failure (compared with 0 percent of health at every size participants).

Given the entire situation surrounding fat, the fat individual is under constant stress—unless they chose to reject society's current belief system on fat. This stress, in turn, can affect the health of the fat individual.

Fat individuals often have everything blamed on their fat. Fall, a commenter on the blog *Dead of Winter,* noted the frustration fat individuals face when attempting to deal with life in general: "Everyone is allowed to have health problems and family problems and emotional problems, except me. I just have fat problems, somehow."

The correlations that do exist between fat and health issues have been used as an excuse to oppress and demean fat people, making health issues for the fat individual even worse. Our current approaches to these health issues have been ineffectual at best and harmful at worst. Maybe we should try a new approach to fat.

not true for all of population, people do believe and trust the system.

# Chapter 6
## It's Not About Health, It's About Money

Looking at the evidence, if we accept that fat is not the problem we hear it is, that dieting does not work, and that the "obesity epidemic" is not the problem we have been led to believe, then why is the medical establishment so determined to demonize fat?

Perhaps the largest source of fuel for fat prejudice is that weight loss is such a lucrative business—one that needs to show little or no results in order to make large amounts of money, Gina Kolata writes in *Rethinking Thin*. By stating that "obesity" itself was a disease—rather than a genetic characteristic or an effect of other factors such as illness or prescription drugs—a number of groups were able to profit in some way from trying to contain that disease.

In 2009, MarketData Enterprises estimated that dieting and weight loss made a $60.9 billion industry—a great deal of money for a product that fails the vast majority of the time. To put this number in perspective, the same company estimates that the U.S. medical laboratories market makes $47 billion a year.

Campos calls "obesity" the "ideal disease," saying that it "never killed those who suffered from it...could not be treated effectively, and...doctors and their patients would nevertheless insist on treating anyway." In "The Politics of Pathology: How Obesity Became an Epidemic Disease," Eric Oliver claims that a number of people profited from labeling "obesity" as a disease:

> Weight-loss doctors use the disease model to promote their business: once you can label fat people as "sick," then it is easy to convince them and their insurers they need treatment and medication. Government health agencies, such as the CDC, are under continual budget pressure, and they sustain their budget allocations by convincing their primary "customer" (Congress) that the nation has a real health problem. Thus, they inflate the number of deaths and the severity of illness that result from increased weight. Academic obesity researchers and scientists often exaggerate or play up the dire impact of obesity to help them secure more research funding, heighten the importance of their own work, or advance their own political causes.

In one interview, Linda Bacon noted that "Fear-mongering about weight is worth billions to industry and is consistent with government policy. Few stand to gain from the news that "overweight" is benign, if not beneficial."

Pharmaceutical companies also have a great stake in trying to make people thin. "A diet pill is a nearly perfect product," Oliver says, since "anyone who wanted to stay thin by using a diet drug would have to stay on the medication perpetually," producing a lifetime customer.

Of course, we have seen this medicalization—that is, as Peter Conrad argues in *The Medicalization of Society*, "when nonmedical problems become defined and treated as medical problems"—of natural human functions and natural human diversity for the sake of money before, with pregnancy and infertility, says Elizabeth Britt, as well as with menopause, baldness and erectile dysfunction, says Conrad. With everyone from pharmaceutical companies to government agencies to academics getting funding out of the need to eradicate fat, "obesity" is definitely a moneymaker.

The anti-fat industry appears to be well aware of the profitability of dieting. Seeing the profitability of the diet rollercoaster for white women, the diet industry started targeting other populations. In the 1990s a study published in *Pediatrics* noted that African American women were more comfortable with their size, even though they tended to be larger than white women. Government agencies and the diet industry saw this as a new market even before the study was released, Laura Fraser says. The DMPI then specifically targeted these populations, trying to get them on the diet-lose-gain-more-diet rollercoaster. In another instance men became the target, in a 1995 campaign by Weight Watchers—again, with the purpose of starting them on the same dysfunctional cycle. Personally, I believe that the entire hype of the "obesity epidemic" came in some portion from the DMPI. Of course, the American people took the bait and ran with it. Do I have proof? Not directly, no. I have not tracked down every article and every move behind the epidemic. However, each time I can trace the source of the messages, I find a pharmaceutical company in some way connected to the original message.

We may not be able to find definitive proof, but we can look at the connections. What we do know is that the International Obesity Task Force (IOTF) is behind the change in definitions for "overweight" and "obesity" that instigated the "obesity epidemic." We know William H. Dietz, an anti-"obesity" crusader and employee of the CDC, is associated with the IOTF. We also know the IOTF is funded primarily by pharmaceutical companies. These facts are pointed out in a *British Medical Journal* article by Ray Moynihan entitled "Obesity task force linked to WHO takes 'millions' from drug firms."

The IOTF is behind a great deal of the research that is being used to justify the war on fat today, which means that pharmaceutical companies are behind many of the messages we receive about fat—an industry that has much to gain by the diet rollercoaster. Additionally, *New York Times* writer Duff Wilson says as many as eight members of the nineteen-member federal panel on "obesity" are "taking money in various forms from companies that could profit from their recommendations." Donna H. Ryan, M.D., co-chairwoman of the "obesity" panel, received payment from companies with a financial interest in the panel's decisions. Duff points out the conflicts:

> GlaxoSmithKline, maker of Alli, an over-the-counter product, has made payments to four of [the federal "obesity" panel members]. Four have financial ties to Allergan, maker of the Lap-Band stomach device. One is paid to speak or advise 11 companies with obesity products. And others consult for companies like Nestlé or Weight Watchers.

These connections are the ones we know about; I suspect many more exist under the table. Such connections guarantee that those with a financial interest in hating fat are making our federal guidelines on "obesity" and are producing our research. So how can we trust such information? To put it simply, we can't.

When those funding the research have so much to gain from a particular outcome, researchers do have the tendency to adjust their research methods to provide such outcomes (see De Vries, Anderson & Martinson's *Journal of Empirical Research on Human Research Ethics* article "Normal Misbehavior: Scientists Talk About the Ethics of Research" for a more in-depth examination of this phenomena). As Gina Kolata says:

> But when your support, and your money, comes from making sure that the growing number of "obese" and overweight people is a major public health priority, there may be at least subtle pressures to emphasize the dire consequence of weight gain and the importance of los-

ing weight, whether or not the science fully backs those claims.

Dieting is big business. And keeping the money rolling in means keeping the fat-negative messages coming.

Participants in the Fatosphere often voice frustration with the monetary implications of weight control. Meowser claims that even the junk food industry profits from diet mania: "half the shit they make wouldn't be half as appetizing to people if they didn't think they weren't 'supposed' to be eating it, nor would nearly as many binge-sized portions of it be consumed." Companies seem to be very aware of the connection between dieting and junk food eating, considering that Weight Watchers has teamed up with McDonald's while Nestlé bought Jenny Craig. Like other nonmedical situations that have been medicalized for the sake of monetary gain, weight loss and dieting have become focuses simply as a means to generate income.

These industries have a great deal of interest in keeping the American public hating fat. They have, in fact, encouraged the oppression of and prejudice toward fat individuals, whether they meant to or not. I would not be surprised to find out that the DMPI set out to increase such prejudice just to increase profits. Since fat individuals are facing oppression and are told that in order to quit being oppressed they must lose weight, they are likely to respond with desperation, grasping at any possible solution—as we see in American society's current situation regarding fat. This desperation significantly expands the profits of those businesses providing weight loss "solutions."

This situation, once again, leads the fat person to the Sisyphean bind—lose weight to be acceptable, gain back more, lose it again, gain again, *ad infinitum*. All the while fat individuals blame themselves for the failure. What an amazing product!

It is time for us to recognize the harm this focus on fat is doing, both to the fat individual and our society itself, all in the name of profit.

# The Attraction of Weight Loss

WEIGHT LOSS IS VERY ATTRACTIVE, ALMOST ADDICTIVE, AND the weight loss industry knows this—hence Weight Watchers encouraging individuals to lose just 10 percent. Since many individuals have seen the failure of diets and are less willing to spend money on expensive diet programs—as exemplified by LA Weight Loss going out of business—the diet industry has once again started losing profits. So to make sure individuals continue weight cycling they have now started pushing for small losses—once again, a brilliant rhetorical move by the DMPI.

When people lose weight, they tend to do so by eating better and exercising, a situation that usually makes people feel better whether they lose weight or not. In her HAES study, Linda Bacon proved that eating better and exercising can improve health whether or not an individual lost weight, so better health outcomes are not surprising. Individuals tend to feel better after only a little weight loss because they tend to treat their bodies better while pursuing weight loss. Additionally, with our society so focused on weight loss, those who lose weight often get complimented and fawned over. Hirschmann and Munter say that such desire for more weight loss is actually a desire to be a different person, a fantasy person with different needs, and weight loss triggers this fantasy.

This is the thing: We have a tendency to fool ourselves. We tell ourselves it's for our health. However, if that were true, then the HAES approach would actually be a better option. We tell ourselves we only want to lose 10 percent. I have found that I don't want to stop until I'm what society thinks is perfect. A little weight loss almost always leads to the desire for more. And the diet industry has figured this out, using arguments suggesting only a little weight loss to keep people on the dieting cycle.

# Chapter 7
## It's Not About Health, It's About Manipulation

**Medical research provides *ethos* (credibility) to the oppression of** fat individuals. Though I have provided a great deal of evidence based in scientific studies to combat the current beliefs regarding fat, these claims can be refuted with the many studies that are in some way fat-negative. Study after study has come out showing how fat bad is, how we need to lose weight, how fat is going to kill us. Yet at closer examination, many of these studies reach their conclusions through questionable means. We want to believe in science; we want to believe that our scientists are unbiased and principled and are really trying to find out the real situation. However, in many instances surrounding fat, reality simply isn't the case.

In American society, we tend to associate research with a search for accuracy, with a way to find solid, believable answers, a way to find Truth with a capital "T." We toss off the words "research says" as if we are imparting laws of nature and the universe. We have privileged this type of information, giving it ethos and power in our daily choices from whether or not we eat eggs to how we teach our children. And for-profit companies have recognized this tendency in the American people, making sure that research shows results that will increase the company's profits.

Through the last few decades more and more research has been debunked because of fraudulent or faulty methodology, leading us to question the validity of what we are told. Thomson Reuters found that published medical studies have increased 44 percent percent since 2001, yet refuted medical studies have increased 15-fold—22 refuted studies in 2001, 139 in 2006, and 339 in 2010. In fact, a 2011 study by medical ethics researcher Grant Steen has shown a steep increase in fraudulent medical research overall.

The reality is that much of our science has been manipulated to get particular results. A researcher makes many, many decisions that may skew the end results. Even researchers who are attempting to be unbiased are likely to have bias creep into their work. So it can be pretty easy for the researcher to manipulate the outcomes toward a particular bias, even when not meaning to. And those researchers who want a particular result can usually find a way to manipulate their methods in order to prove something in particular. Whether it be from questionable assumptions, faulty research methods or out-and-out fraud, we need to question any research we see—but most especially research that can lead to profit.

## Questionable Assumptions

EVEN WHEN RESEARCHERS ARE HONESTLY TRYING TO GET AT the truth, many studies are based on faulty assumptions at best and out-and-out prejudice at worst. Many "obesity" researchers approach their research with the assumption that fat individuals are fat because of habits, a belief that has been repeatedly proven incorrect, as noted before. These assumptions underlie so much of the research and medical practices associated with "obesity," and are incredibly harmful because they set the researcher up to ask the wrong questions. When a researcher believes that eating too much is the problem, they look for ways to make fat people eat less. Such approaches then lead to solutions such as weight loss surgery, which often leaves the fat individual malnourished, as researcher Scott Malinowski has found.

Let's consider the way we talk about the increase in weight in the U.S. The increase in the incidence of "overweight" and "obese" is often cited as reason for concern, the reason for the "obesity epidemic." For instance, Rokholm et al. said in a *Public Library of Science ONE* article about genetic variance and "obesity" that "There is no doubt that the dramatic worldwide increase in obesity prevalence is due to changes in environmental factors." Actually, a great deal of doubt exists on whether or not we even have much of an increase in "obesity" (see Linda Bacon's book *Health At Every Size* for a thorough deconstruction of that argument), let alone what has caused the slight increase we can track. Yet this assumption of Rokholm et al.'s colored their entire study, making their conclusions suspect.

Because these researchers make faulty assumptions, they will then have faulty research. Some of this mismanagement is purposeful, in the case of DMPI-funded research trying to keep people in the weight loss/regain cycle. Some of these researchers truly want to help fat individuals and believe their assumptions, considering the depth of societal prejudice. However, such assumptions make much of "obesity" research inaccurate or out-and-out invalid. As medical consumers, we must always question the assumptions of any research we take into consideration.

## *Everyone Knows*

THE PREDOMINANT MESSAGE WE RECEIVE ABOUT FAT MAKES it sound as if the medical community is united on the ideas that fat is unhealthy and changeable and that fat individuals must be either educated or coerced into weight loss. Actually, a great deal of controversy exists in the medical community regarding this belief. Laura Fraser argues that this controversy comes from "obesity" researchers holding conflicting points of view—"pro-diet medical researchers and anti-diet eating disorders researchers." Additionally, she asserts, these camps interpret data in very different ways. I believe we also have a split between those researchers who are just trying to please their funders and those who are trying to generate research that is as non-biased as possible.

To illustrate this controversy, I examined three medical articles detailing studies of "obesity" tied to longevity and the medical communities' reaction to these studies: two studies revealing the dangers of "obesity" and one showing the protective qualities of "obesity." By looking at these studies in detail, we can see how the medical community handles such controversy.

In 1999 Allison, Fontaine, Manson, Stevens, and VanItallie published an article in *JAMA* entitled "Annual Deaths Attributable to Obesity in the United States." The authors were attempting to determine how many deaths could be attributed to "obesity" each year.

Allison and his team used a formula much like the conventional attributable risk formulae, but accounting for "complications." The overall population of the study consisted of individuals 18 years or older within the U.S. The actual data from the study came from a number of sources including the Alameda County Health Study, the Framingham Heart Study, the Tecumseh Community Health Study, the American Cancer Society Cancer Prevention Study I, the Nurses' Health Study, and the National Health and Nutrition Examination Survey (NHANES) I. For the actual statistical process of the study, Allison et al. started with the Cox proportional hazards regression model, using dummy codes for BMI categories as defined by the covariate age and sex, as well as defining dummy codes for smoking status. In general, however, the authors ignored the covariates, since they were trying to look at the general population overall. Allison and his team chose to keep early deaths in the ratio. They ran the numbers with both smokers and nonsmokers.

The researchers found that the risks increased with the increase in BMI, and at the reference level, higher BMI actually had "protective" qualities. They also found that for never-smokers the numbers were even higher for higher BMI categories. The authors do note that this study does not take into account "confounding from other sources (e.g., prevalent chronic disease, unintentional weight loss, weight fluctuation)."

The second study I looked at, entitled "Excess Deaths Associated with Underweight, Overweight and Obesity" by Katherine Flegal and a team of medical researchers supported by the Centers for Disease Control, was published in *JAMA* in April 2005. This article detailed a research project that considered levels of BMI and the risks of mortality. The authors reported that "obese" individuals (individuals with a BMI greater than 30) were connected with 111,909 excess deaths; "underweight" individuals (individuals with a BMI less than 18.5) were associated with 33,746 excess deaths; and "overweight" individuals (individuals with a BMI greater than 25 and less than 30) were actually associated with a reduction in deaths— -86,094 compared to those individuals considered "normal" weight. The researchers used a standard statistical survival model called the Cox proportional hazard model on the results of three different NHANE surveys covering 1971 to 1994. Flegal et al. explained that they ran the numbers many times using a variety of models and taking a variety of factors into account, such as smoking and weight loss caused by illness. They provided tables of this data online and concluded that these factors had no major impact on the estimates.

The final article I considered, "Overweight, Obesity, and Mortality in a Large Prospective Cohort of Persons 50 to 71 Years Old" by Adams et al., was published in the *New England Journal of Medicine* in 2006. In this study the authors sought to determine whether or not "overweight" was associated with a higher risk of death. Adams et al. used information from the National Institutes of Health-American Association of Retired Persons (NIH-AARP) Diet and Health Study, including a supplemental questionnaire requesting self-reported weights from as many as 20 years earlier. This study was developed by the National Cancer Institute in order "to improve our understanding of the relationship between diet and health." This team of investigators found many similarities to Flegal et al.'s findings, and some significant differences.

Adams et al. found that the highest risks did lie at the statistical extremes of weight—those with the highest and the lowest BMIs—much like Flegal's team found. These investigators then considered each covariate, including smoking status and preexisting disease, in relation to "obesity." Adams determined that excess weight accounted for about 18 percent of premature deaths in never-smokers—18.1 percent of men and 18.7 percentt of women. In discussing the results, the authors note that "obesity was strongly associated with the risk of death in both men and women in all racial and ethnic groups and at all ages," and that even small increases in BMI increased the danger of death.

Though these three articles looked at the same concept—how "overweight" and "obesity" affects longevity—they did so in very different ways, using very different methods. There were problems and positives with all of the studies.

Allison et al. used very old data from six distinctly different data sets, some of which contained self-reported information. Additionally, they correlated particular diseases to "overweight" and "obesity," then claimed that everyone who died of that disease counted as a death caused by "obesity." These researchers did, however, look at a great deal of data in the process of their study.

Flegal and her team appeared to use a very complicated statistical process in the course of their research. On the other hand, they explained their process in detail. Additionally, they used very reliable data gleaned through the NHANES.

Adams et al. used self-reported data, some of which was remembered from as much as twenty years earlier. Additionally, this data was primarily from white, middle- or upper-class and educated individuals—a poor representation of our overall population. At the same time, these researchers had a very large data set to work from.

In responding to these articles, the medical community questioned the methods of both those who supported the dominant rhetoric and those who did not. Flegal's team as well as Adams et al. had their articles closely examined by experts in the field—experts who found fault with the researchers' process. A team of M.D.s led by Walter C. Willett, chair of Harvard's Department of Nutrition, stated that Flegal et al.'s "analysis does not successfully disentangle" lower weight individuals who are "a mix of smokers, healthy active persons, and those with chronic illness." Specifically, Willett et al. state that Flegal's team never considered those with weight loss previous to baseline at the same time as those who never smoked. Willett's group goes on to use previous studies to argue that "overweight" individuals have a number of problems that lead to life-threatening diseases, therefore Flegal et al.'s information must be in error.

Ding, a member of the Department of Epidemiology at the Harvard School of Public Health, questioned Flegal and her team's use of a proportional hazard model and suggested instead a random-effects model. Another group of M.D.s led by Strickler questioned the use of the BMI as a gauge. Greenberg,

a Ph.D. from the Department of Health and Nutrition Sci-
ences at Brooklyn College, argued that Flegal's team did not
take two confounders into account—that elderly persons tend
to lose weight before dying and the potential "regression-to-
the-mean patterns in the BMI data." In an editorial printed
in the same issue as Flegal's original article, Mark, a contrib-
uting editor to *JAMA*, questioned whether "obesity" can even
be studied, and suggested instead that researchers focus on the
benefits of diet and exercise programs.

These attacks proved to be too little for Willett. For some
reason (most likely financial connections to the DMPI), he
needed to out-and-out attack Flegal et al. First, instead of a scientific study, the Harvard School of Public Health responded
with a survey showing that Americans still thought "obesity"
was a problem:

> The past year has seen scientific studies that have var-
> ied in their estimates of the seriousness of obesity and
> overweight and their impact on premature death. A new
> opinion poll by the Harvard School of Public Health
> finds that most Americans have not changed their minds
> about the seriousness of the obesity problem and do
> not believe that scientific experts are overestimating the
> health risks of obesity. In addition, they are no less likely
> than a year ago to be keeping track of calories, fat con-
> tent, or the amount of carbohydrates they eat.

> Three-fourths of Americans rate obesity as an "extreme-
> ly"(34%) or "very"(41%) serious public health problem
> in the United States. In addition, the majority of Ameri-
> cans believe that scientific experts have been portraying
> accurately (58%) or even underestimating (22%) the
> health risks of being obese. Very few Americans reported
> believing that the health risks were being overestimated
> by scientific experts (15%).

Then, as reported in Gina Kolata's book *Rethinking Thin*,
in "an exercise in attack science," a team of "obesity" research-

ers led by Willett held a daylong seminar with the single focus of refuting Flegal et al.'s work—an act unheard of previously. They attacked Flegal et al.'s work for not excluding smokers and those already ill, a point which Flegal said is not true. Even the authors'. credentials as Ph.D.s in nutrition were attacked because they were not M.D.s. As noted in *Rethinking Thin,* Flegal was surprised at just how vehemently her work and her credentials were attacked:

"Everyone thinks they already know the answer," she says. "Anything that doesn't fit, they have to explain it away or ignore it. All these people who just know weight loss is good for you. It's just taken for granted regardless of the evidence."

Research that shows "obesity" is not a large problem definitely receives negative response from the medical community.

However, research supporting the dominant rhetoric is not immune from criticism either. C. Appels and J.P. Vandenbroucke, both M.D.s at Leiden University Medical Center in the Netherlands, criticize Adams et al. for using a study that consisted "mainly of white, highly educated people." They also noted that the response rate, only 18 percent, was poor. Appels and Vandenbroucke claimed that the study resulted in an "immortality bias" because "respondents could not have died between 50 years of age and enrollment." These physicians claimed that all of these factors led to "multiple selection biases."

Another physician, J.H. Hoofnagle of the National Institutes of Health, says that the findings were skewed because of the elimination of those who had smoked, leaving only 30 percent of the original group. Hoofnagle claimed that "the use of relative risks and death rates per 100,000 person-years gives an inflated picture of the differences." This physician claims that the results actually showed only a minimal increased risk for "overweight," never-smoking individuals. U.S. Barzel of the Montefiore Medical Center asserted that the self-reported nature of the weight data results "in some uncertainty in the validity of the actual data." Additionally, Barzel notes, BMI alone is not a valid factor since it does not take into account subcutaneous or abdominal fat. J. Spitzer, a professor at the San Francisco Conservatory of Music, states that unlike Adams et al.'s claim, the population was not from the Baby Boomer generation. Spitzer says that the Baby Boomers were born after August 1945—the end of World War II—and the majority of Adams' cohort was born between 1924 and 1945.

Yet fat studies authors and fat-positive bloggers argue that the medical community does not adequately critique work that finds fat unhealthy, noting that the results are often manipulated. Individuals in both groups have argued that both Allison and Adams et al. manipulated the results of their studies. Eric Oliver argues that Allison's study did not take other explanatory factors "such as genes, diet patterns, or exercise" into account. In addition, he argues that Allison assumed that any excess death in fat individuals was caused by fat. "Even if an obese person died in a car accident or from a snakebite," Oliver argues, "the cause of his or her death was attributed to body weight."

Campos blasted Adams et al.'s research in his weekly opinion column in the *Rocky Mountain News*. He started his column with a tongue-in-cheek comment on the reliability of the study: "Confessions extracted under torture are notoriously unreliable. A new study in *The New England Journal of Medicine* illustrates this point well." Campos went on to say that Adams et al. were so determined to refute Flegal et al.'s finding that they "tortured" the data to get the desired results. He proceeded to step through his view of Adams et al.'s manipulations of the data, saying that throwing out all smokers did not lead to the desired conclusion, so the authors, rather than using the participants' current weight, used a self-reported weight from age 50. Campos claimed that Adams et al. finally found their desired results using these self-reported numbers: that those who were "overweight" at 50 and "normal weight" when they entered the study had a marginal increase in mortality. Campos ended his column by stating that, when read closely, the study actually refutes the desired results; however, the journalists reporting this information will not be able to figure that out because Adams hid it so well.

Bacon was quoted in *The Washington Post* as saying that she believed "the researchers were trying to manipulate their data to match their conclusion." Bacon says that Adams et al. found the same result as Flegal et al., so they "subjected their data to numerous manipulations before finally arriving at a suitable conclusion." She notes that they discarded all data on smokers or former smokers. When that did not support their conclusion, they used only a portion of the "normal weight" group in comparison with the entire "overweight" group. When that did not support their desired outcome, Bacon claims, they then asked individuals what they weighed at 50. Since some of these individuals were in their 70s at the time and 40 percent of the participants did not answer the question, Bacon argued that the information was probably not accurate.

Finally, Bacon lists a number of other reasons the information was weak: a low response rate that is not representative of the nation as a whole; self-reported data; poorly constructed adjustments of potential confounders; and finally that "weight loss is associated with a significant increased risk of death for middle-aged 'overweight' people." Bacon concludes by accusing the *New England Journal of Medicine* of providing propaganda rather than scholarship.

Though the medical establishment only accused Flegal et al. of poor research methods, the body acceptance movement accuses Adams' team of out-and-out data manipulation in order to get the specific desired results.

Both Adams' and Flegal's teams have been accused of poor

research methods that have led to inaccurate results. Is this a situation where rivals are simply trying to debunk information that does not support their points of view? Since these groups' beliefs are foundationally oppositional, this may well be the case. Because each group holds such bias, any results supporting their points of view must be viewed as somewhat suspect.

One note for consideration: Flegal and her team actually appear to support the dominant medical rhetoric. Though they do argue for their findings, they appear almost uncomfortable with the results. That may give more credence to the findings of this study than to the Adams et al. study that supports the dominant view. Either way, we can see that though the dominant culture more readily supports studies that sustain the status quo, controversy definitely exists within the medical community itself.

Though the examination of these three articles provided a very small slice of the medical rhetoric surrounding "obesity," it does appear that the medical community is not willing to support research simply because it sustains the status quo—though they do tend to be harder on studies that suggest fat is not associated with disease in itself. This look at three articles provides only a small step in understanding how the medical community handles controversy within its midst, especially controversy that questions the common belief systems of the dominant beliefs. However, this limited project gives us a glimpse into the complex world of medical rhetoric. If nothing else, it reveals the depth and breadth of attitudes within the medical community. Though there may be a dominant belief system within this group, that belief system is not held by all. While there may be a common train of thought, there are those who are willing to consider research that does not support it.

# When All Else Fails: Lie

WHEN CONSIDERING FAULTY RESEARCH METHODS, ONE OF-
ten thinks of high profile cases involving very unethical behavior such as falsification, fabrication, and plagiarism. At least
one incident of such behavior exists in anti-"obesity" research.

The belief that fat is unhealthy is so prevalent in the medical field that when his research did not reveal a connection
between "obesity" and sleep apnea, Robert B. Fogel, M.D., a
former professor at Harvard's medical school, falsified the data.
The Office of Research Integrity reports that Fogel:

- Changed/falsified roughly half of the physiologic data.

- Fabricated roughly 20 percent of the anatomic data that
  were supposedly obtained from Computed Tomography
  (CT) images.

- Changed/falsified 50 to 80 percent of the other anatomic
  data.

- Changed/falsified roughly 40 to 50 percent of the sleep data
  so that those data would better conform to his hypothesis.

- Respondent also published some of the falsified and fabricated data in an abstract in *Sleep* 24, Abstract Supplement
  A7, 2001.

Fogel may have had financial reasons to fabricate his data.
Though this research was funded by the National Institutes of
Health, Fogel had close ties to the pharmaceutical industry. In
fact, by the time this research misbehavior came to light, Fogel
was working for Merck, a pharmaceutical company.

The fact that Fogel's true data showed that sleep apnea is not
connected to "obesity" has been ignored by the medical com-

munity. For instance, the National Heart, Lung, and Blood Institute states on its "obesity" education page that "reducing the prevalence of overweight will help reduce the prevalence and severity of sleep apnea."

In such cases as Fogel's, there is little question that research is being manipulated and polished to receive a particular result. However, though no one knows exactly how often such falsified studies happen, in the *Journal of Empirical Research on Human Research Ethics* de Vries et al. suggest they appear to be relatively rare in today's scientific community. What is more common are the little ways in which scientists consciously or unconsciously manipulate data in order to receive the answer they were searching for.

In a 2005 article on "Good Research Conduct" in the *Archives of Disease in Childhood*, Jonathan Grigg, M.D. argues that even conscientious researchers must be aware of the potential to perform bad research. He specifically considers problems such as duplicate publication, conflict of interest, authorship, and data storage, and explains why rules about research conduct are so important:

> [I]t may seem that bureaucracy and rules exist to get in the way of, rather than to enable, clinical research. However, the presence of these rules and their complexity exist because clinical researchers have a unique responsibility to both science and patients.

Even a conscientious researcher may be crafting results if they are not aware of potential problems in the research process.

Less conscientious researchers are even more likely to manipulate results. Subtle research misbehavior occurs on a regular basis.

Using a set of anonymous surveys developed from a series of focus groups, sociologists Brian C. Martinson, Melissa S. Anderson and Raymond de Vries sought to quantify such "normal misbehaviors" among scientists. Though less publicized than falsification, fabrication, and plagiarism, these "normal misbehaviors" are "more common and more worrisome to researchers, if less visible to the public," Martinson et al. say. Though few scientists—only 0.3 percent—admitted to "cooking" or falsification of data, a full 15.5 percent admitted to "changing the design, methodology or results of a study in response to pressure from a funding source." The same survey revealed that 10.8 percent of scientists withheld "details of methodology or results in papers or proposals," while 13.5 percent admitted to "using inadequate or inappropriate research designs."

Martinson et al. suggest that the number of "misbehaving scientists" actually may be quite a bit higher than their study found, since scientists engaging in such behavior may be unwilling to respond to such a survey.

These numbers imply that a significant percentage of researchers do use research methodology to get the answers they desire rather than to simply determine what is really going on. These manipulations may be as little as a failing to present data that conflicts with their own desired results or as big as cooking data. Whichever it is, a number of scientists are self-admittedly crafting the results of their research projects.

Given that much of the funding for research surrounding fat comes from pharmaceutical companies and the diet industry, finding positive aspects to fat can be detrimental to a researcher's funding options. "Researchers who oppose dieting don't stand much of a change of getting funding from companies who know the research will undermine their products," Fraser writes.

Since scientists often change their method or methodology to please their funders, in considering the work of "obesity" researchers it helps to understand their affiliations. Looking at the authors of the three earlier articles, we can see that affiliations may indeed have an effect on research outcomes.

For the Allison et al. article, both David B. Allison, Ph.D. and Theodore B. VanItallie, M.D. are researchers at the Obesity Research Center at St. Luke's/Roosevelt Hospital Center; the rest of the authors (Kevin R. Fontaine, Ph.D., JoAnn E. Manson, M.D., Dr.Ph. & June Stevens, Ph.D.) are associated with academic departments. With the exception of Stevens, all of these researchers have financial ties to the weight loss industry, with Allison having "received grants, honoraria, monetary and product donations, was a consultant to, and had contracts or other commitments with numerous organizations involving weight control products and services."

Considering the Flegal et al. study: Katherine M. Flegal, Ph.D. works out of the National Center for Health Statistics, a division of the CDC, as well as the Center for Weight and Health at the University of California at Berkeley. Barry I. Graubard, Ph.D. and Mitchell H. Gail, M.D., Ph.D. are associated with the Division of Cancer Epidemiology and Genetics, a part of the National Cancer Institute. David F. Williamson, Ph.D. is also with the CDC, though in the Division of Diabetes Translation. These researchers have no known connections to the weight loss or pharmaceutical industries.

Basically, we can't fully trust research. But not trusting research can lead us into quite a bind. How do we find solutions if we can't trust research as a guide?

The first step, I believe, is to quite privileging research just because it has an air of science.

Be critical of studies. Look at what other experts say about the research. When considering a research study, if you can, find out where the funding for the research comes from. Consider the affiliations of the researchers as well as their assumptions and attitudes. If you cannot find these things out, test the research against what you have found in your own life or what other individuals have experienced in theirs. In my experience, finding out the experience of a person tends to help me make decisions more than research does.

We don't want to throw research completely away; however, we can't just believe what researchers say, either. We must be critical consumers of research, especially when making a decision that may affect our health.

# Chapter 8
## It's Not About Health, It's About Morality

We want to think the "obesity epidemic" is about health; however, we cannot ignore the moral outrage that has been generated by the idea that fat people must become thin. Paul Campos and others call the furor over the "obesity epidemic" a "moral panic." Campos explains how this moral panic works:

> First, a group or behavior is classified as dangerously deviant. The deviance is characterized as both a serious threat to societal welfare and as a symptom of deep social ills. The media whips up public concern on the subject by focusing rapidly increasing amounts of attention on it, often in an alarmist fashion that exaggerates the extent of—and the danger presented by—the behavior and those who engage in it. This in turn leads decision makers to act, usually with the stated goal of completely eliminating, or at least greatly reducing, the deviants and/or their behavior. Whether or not the action is successful, the panic eventually recedes as public attention moves on to other threats, real or imagined.

The situation surrounding fat in the U.S. definitely fits this concept of a moral panic.

On the surface, making everyone fit the "normal" weight

range seems to be about making everyone the same. Rhetorician Elizabeth Britt sees the norm as "an argument about what is desirable." Britt says normalization itself seeks to "identify the normal and the abnormal" while attempting to reform the abnormal.

In reality, however, the push for normality hides the real goal of finding a scapegoat. Michel Foucault, a rhetorician and philosopher, notes the function of normalization and the discipline used to enforce that normalization "is not intended to eliminate offenses," but rather to differentiate the compliant from the noncompliant. In this disciplinary system that searches to normalize all individuals, "bodies are individually and minutely observed, their activities measured, and their measurements compared and averaged," says Britt. "Those individuals falling outside desirable values," she argues, "are subjected to reform"— a fitting description of the current situation with the "obesity epidemic."

Fat has been labeled as "deviant" in our society, and in return it appears that society seeks to normalize the fat individual—to make everyone fall within a certain weight range. The truth is much less appetizing. Rather than seeking to make everyone the same, this dynamic is actually striving to establish the "good" folks from the "bad" folks.

These attempts to control peoples' weights, this disciplinary system, provide a potent example of what Foucault calls "bio-power." Foucault defines bio-power as "an explosion of numerous and diverse techniques for achieving the subjugation of bodies and the control of populations." In other words, bio-power is a force that establishes understood truths about bodies that, after being internalized, take on normalizing and regulatory functions, often working to oppress individuals—a point argued by the rhetoricians Blake Scott and Jeannette Herrle-Fanning. Rhetorician Mary Lay says this power establishes and legitimizes authorities who create and perpetuate "a distinction between the normal and abnormal." These authorities establish a binary system—"licit and illicit, permitted and forbidden," asserts Foucault. This type of power does not impose itself from without, but rather creates a need within the individual to meet the norms. Lay says that experts—"individuals who successfully claim "authoritative knowledge"—start representing bio-power and, using the influence of bio-power combined with authoritative knowledge, start creating a framework for control.

The conventional point of view toward fat has taken on the guise of authoritative knowledge—that is, knowledge that carries influence because of its efficacy in explaining the state of the world or because of its association with a stronger power base (structural superiority), or usually both, says scholar B. Jordan. "Obesity" experts claim authoritative knowledge in the realm of our beliefs regarding fat. These experts are often very biased against fat individuals, as noted previously, and have a personal incentive for keeping fat hatred rampant—they earn their living attempting to eradicate fat. This authoritative knowledge becomes the language of the dominant message since it is highly valued.

According to a group of rhetoricians led by Lay, another aspect to authoritative knowledge includes the fact that other systems of knowledge are silenced or devalued. As Bernadette Longo, Ph.D. said, "Devalued knowledge, like a counterfeit coin, will not circulate widely in this economy; highly valued knowledge will circulate widely as the genuine coin." People then begin "to see this social order as the natural order, adding to the persuasive power of authoritative knowledge," argues Lay and colleagues.

So by the very nature of authoritative knowledge, knowledge that sees fat as benign such as the HAES paradigm will be devalued. Diet books and the like take on the appearance of authoritative knowledge, giving the oppression of fat individuals social power.

Scientific and medical communication play a part in this normalization process by "legitimating and subjugating knowledges, examining and controlling workplace practices, forming subjectivities, and marking bodies as normal or deviant," says Jason Palmeri, a technical communication scholar.

When we give diet books credence, our society marks the fat individual as deviant.

# The Cost of Being Fat

ANOTHER IMPRESSIVE RHETORICAL MOVE BY THE DMPI WAS to emphasize the costs of "obesity" in health care. Even if fat individuals are unhealthy, however, why should that matter to others?

Exaggerating and even fabricating the costs of "obesity" to the health care system has given thinner individuals the sense of the right to police fat folk, because they see fat as costing them money through Medicare/Medicaid and insurance costs. For example, in a debate entitled "Is it OK to be fat?" MeMe Roth, a vocal anti-"obesity" proponent often quoted or interviewed as an "obesity expert," claimed that thin people experience prejudice because they are expected to pay for "obese" individuals' lifestyle choices.

Because of our systems of Medicaid and insurance, to some degree health care costs are shared by all. Rising health care costs are often blamed on fat individuals. However, such statistics often contain the costs of trying to reduce fat, including the costs of bariatric surgery and diet programs as well as the more insidious costs of medical fat prejudice. As Ragen Chastain says, "let's remember that 'costs of obesity' are not the same as costs of obesity hysteria."

Thus, for instance, when examining a study that claims "obese" children cost more than "normal weight" children,

Sandy Szwarc at the *Junkfood Science* blog noted that the $172 extra costs are caused by physicians requiring more tests of "obese" than of "normal weight" children. Finkelstein emphasized the fact that much of the costs of "obesity" comes from Medicare and Medicaid—not surprising, since many fat individuals come from minority or poverty stricken groups. In my rhetorical analysis of blogs, puellapiscea, a member of the Fatosphere, suggests how these rhetorics of cost and health care contribute to the demand that the individual lose weight:

> Fat, unlike a big nose, or eyes too close together, is ALL MY FAULT. And it isn't just a hurting me (cuz you know fat is unhealthy). With the so-called obesity epidemic I am hurting everyone else with my strain on the health care system. That is a lot more societal punishment and stigma than my frizzy hair ever got.

The medical establishment has made an individual's fat body other people's issue by conflating the costs of fat, saying that "obesity" is costing the general public more in terms of insurance and health care costs. This rhetorical action is yet another move that legitimizes fat prejudice. Now fat people have a moral obligation to get thin so they don't cost others money.

## Smoking, Drinking & Obesity

IN ANOTHER MOVE THAT PLACES FAT IN THE "IMMORAL" CATegory, "obesity" is often compared to smoking, drugging and drinking. "Obesity," a body size—not a behavior—is often placed in the same noncompliant category as such unhealthy behaviors. For example, in the book *Doctors Talking with Patients/Patients Talking with Doctors: Improving Communication in Medical Visits* by Debra L. Roter and Judith A. Hall, the authors lump "weight control" in with smoking cessation, alcohol restriction and other lifestyle changes. Even "obesity" expert Arya Sharma, M.D. has gotten into the mix by comparing fat activists to smoking advocates on his blog.

We can find many problems with placing "obesity" in the same category as addiction. First off, we must consider the language issues—as in parts of speech. As a teacher of writing, I must point out that smoking and drinking are verbs, while "obesity" is a noun; smoking and drinking are actions, while "obesity" is a state of being. Jay Solomon, founder of the More of Me to Love online community, says the equivalent of "smoking" for fat people would be "obesing"—not a real world.

Fat is a very different thing than addiction. Behavior is not the same thing as a body characteristic. Individuals can stop drinking or smoking for a day; they cannot just stop being fat for a day. Yet our society tends to believe that "obesity" is an outward sign of behavior—an argument I have already debunked in Chapter 4. So society lumps body size in with addiction, setting up a faulty premise for ineffectual health care interventions.

Placing "obese" individuals into this category implies that "obese" persons are fat because of addiction, which simply is not true. Arguing that fat is caused by addiction suggests a single cause behind people being fat—eating too much. Though overeating does exist as a behavioral disorder, we greatly harm both overeaters and fat individuals by assuming all fat individuals eat pathologically and that all compulsive overeaters must be fat. Those who overeat pathologically—no matter their size—need support and help, not moral judgment. (See Chapter 4 for a deeper discussion of eating disorders.)

Additionally, believing that the problem is overeating implies that the fat individual should give up eating. Neither alcohol nor nicotine is needed for daily life, but eating is rather an important factor for health. I hate to tell you, but we are all addicted to food. Yes, without food we would not live, unlike surviving without alcohol or mind-altering drugs.

Some argue that "obesity" is caused by the "soft addiction"—
a term coined by poet Judith Wright—of overeating. Wright
describes soft addictions as "those seemingly harmless habits...
that actually keep us from the life we want." Yet we have already seen that fat is not caused by overeating for the majority
of individuals. So the belief that "obesity" is an external expres-
sion of addiction is foundationally faulty.

By lumping fat individuals in with drug addicts, alcoholics
and smokers, we suggest that fat is, in some way, controllable.
Since some of the most successful ways of controlling alcohol
and drug use are anonymous programs, we cannot really look
at those numbers, but we can look at the success of reducing smoking. The American Heart Association says that "Since
1965, more than 49 percent of all adults who have ever smoked
have quit." That percentage is staggering compared to Mann's
findings that not only do the majority of fat individuals gain
their lost weight back, but at least 82 percent have gained back
all they lost and more by the 2.5 year mark. The current evidence does not support the suggestion that fat is as controllable
as smoking.

Finally, we are living in the 21st century. Haven't we moved
beyond the morality model of addiction? Addiction involves
a very complex combination of factors including genetics
and environment, says the National Institute on Drug Abuse.
Comparing fat to addictive behaviors should not create moral
outrage, but rather a search for a solution. And yet, part of the
reason that many experts have argued to shame fat individuals
is that smoking has decreased through public health campaigns
that use such tactics (for example, see the article by Emery et al.
entitled "Public Health Obesity-Related TV Advertising: Lessons Learned from Tobacco").

So by linking "obesity" to addictive behaviors, our society
tends to think that shaming should reduce "obesity." Yet it
hasn't worked. It hasn't worked because the premise is faulty—

the defective idea that fat is always caused by an energy imbalance, that fat people are fat because they eat too much and exercise too little, that fat people are fat because they are addicted to food. Once again the trope of the out-of-control fat person comes into play, and fat is characterized as a moral issue.

You cannot look at someone and truly know their habits. However, by lumping "obesity" in with unhealthy behaviors, we now have a visual way to judge someone as lacking, as morally wrong. The belief that fat is an outward appearance of addiction has no scientific backing, yet we continue to perpetuate this myth, then insist that fat people get help for their addiction. No wonder interventions toward fat people continue to fail, since the entire premise such interventions are based on is faulty.

# *Healthism*

MAKING FAT A MORAL AFFRONT TO SOCIETY CONTAINS AN ELement of prejudice that we seldom acknowledge in the Western world—healthism. Robert Crawford, the originator of the term, explained healthism in the 1980 article "Healthism and the Medicalization of Everyday Life:"

> Healthism represents a particular way of viewing the health problem, and is characteristic of the new health consciousness and movements. It can best be understood as a form of medicalization, meaning that it still retains key medical notions. Like medicine, healthism situates the problem of health and disease at the level of the individual. Solutions are formulated at that level as well. To the extent that healthism shapes popular beliefs, we will continue to have a non-political, and therefore, ultimately ineffective conception and strategy of health promotion. Further, by elevating health to a super value, a metaphor for all that is good in life, healthism reinforces the privatization of the struggle for generalized well-being.

In other words, as a society we have made it to where you are a "good" person if you are healthy and a "bad" person if you are unhealthy; a state of "health" is morally superior to a state of not being healthy. Since fat is seen as unhealthy whatever a person's actual state of health, fat people are therefore morally "bad."

We can find many issues with healthism itself, but especially with healthism directed toward fat individuals, since healthism is a form of elitism. In the U.S., though some health care may be garnered from the government, good, extensive health care involves money. Because of their lack of access to health care, poor individuals will more likely be unhealthy. With healthism, the individual from a higher socioeconomic bracket may feel morally superior because they may be healthier. Since, as I revealed in Chapter 3, fat individuals are more likely to be of lower socioeconomic standing because of prejudice, healthism can be particularly menacing, producing a nasty cycle—a fat individual gets a lower paying job because of their fat, which leads to poorer healthcare, which may lead to health issues, which can increase fatness.

In our society, individuals can internalize this belief that they are morally bad for being sick. For those who are fat because they are sick or for those who do have diseases that are classed as "obesity related," such as Type 2 diabetes, being sick can feel like a moral failure—being sick makes a fat person a "bad" fat person. Pattie Thomas, Ph.D., a medical sociologist and fat studies scholar, explored this in her blog *FattyPatties:*

> I am aware that a lot of people in the world are cheering at these facts [diabetes, hypothyroidism, post-menopausal] about me, as if they prove something. As if my becoming ill justifies all the weight loss schemes and all the risk factor studies. I am a bad fattie. I am one of those people who supposedly demonstrates that being over 300 pounds means instant death or long-term illness or the absolute end of health care as we know it.

Fat people with health issues can feel like they are bad for being ill. These feelings, along with the health issues, can lead to a strong sense of failure for the fat individual. In turn, these internalized feelings of failure can lead the fat person to accept poor health care or to take desperate, unhealthy measures to procure weight loss.

Deb B goes into detail about the good and bad health paradigm and the pursing of weight loss:

> In fat acceptance circles, we have been talking for decades about the pressure to be a "poster child" for glowing health if we are fat. It's a stereotype management thing. In the eyes of a dubious public, we are split into "good fatty" and "bad fatty" camps depending on whether we eat our vegetables and have normal blood glucose values. When we age and develop the diseases that people across the weight spectrum develop (yes! there are no diseases that only fat people have!), when they are conditions modestly correlated with higher BMI, we feel like we are BUSTED. That emotional experience rocks our faith in our own experience, that dieting has left us with more physical and psychological problems, not less; and we are vulnerable to the "solution" of weight loss because it is scary to get older and less physically resilient. We forget that these experiences of aging happen to everyone—and everyone wants to feel like they have something tangible they can do. Pursuing weight loss is the great global cultural response to just about anything that ails you—and hey, we are all pre-death.

On her blog *The Rotund,* Marianne Kirby argues that we must not equate health and morality:

> health isn't a moral issue. Having a disability doesn't make you a bad fatty or a bad representative of fat acceptance. Taking the stairs doesn't make you a good fatty or a good representative of fat acceptance. And neither make you a good or a bad person.

This statement exemplifies the crux of the matter: We must take morality completely out of the weight picture. Making someone into a "bad fatty," especially when they have no hope of getting "good" (i.e. healthy and thin), doesn't improve anyone's health. It only makes those with such conditions possibly give up. Since the HAES perspective is that anyone's health can get better, shouldn't we use this approach instead?

# Chapter 9
# It's Not About Health,
# It's About Using & Abusing Children

One of the strongest and most compelling cries in the "obesity epidemic" is "but what about the children?" Yes, what about the children? We often hear about the dangers of allowing children to get fat—as if we have a choice. In fact, arguments are appearing in the media suggesting that allowing a child to become fat is a form of child abuse. Children such as Annamarie Regino have been taken away from their parents, later to be given back when foster families had no better luck making them thin. In a commentary in a 2011 issue of *JAMA*, Murtagh and Ludwig argue that severely "obese" children should be taken away from their parents rather than be subjected to bariatric surgery. As Marilyn Wann pointed out in a blog post on *SF Weekly*, Ludwig makes the logical fallacy of a false dichotomy, that there are only two choices. We have many other choices in dealing with health, primarily the HAES approach. Jackie, commenting on *Two Whole Cakes,* makes an interesting observation regarding this practice:

> It seems to me that this "take the children away and fix them" approach has been used over and over again by modern societies to reform socially deviant attributes and behavior.* In the past black children from Australia

to Germany have been institutionalized to civilize them. Although lacking state intervention, gay children are sent to "reform" camps where they will be retrained. It seems only logical that fat children would become another group of deviants to be controlled and reformed. And it's always for the best interest of the child!

Once again, fat people are experiencing oppression based on the assumption of eating too much—that the child is fat because of eating wrong in some way. As exemplified in the case of Annamarie Regino, who was found to have genetic issues, severely "obese" children don't tend to get that way only by what they eat. Yet rather than work with the parents to find out what is truly going on, authorities try to take the children away. In response, parents try harder and harder to make their fat children thin, most likely only making them fatter in the long run.

Fat children are considered such a call for alarm that even the First Lady, Michelle Obama, has gotten into the fray with her "Let's Move" campaign, blaming the U.S.'s economic problems on childhood "obesity." The "Let's Move" website says the campaign focuses on eating healthy and getting active. When fat activists and scholars argue against the campaign, they are not arguing against the idea that children should be encouraged to exercise and eat well—they are arguing that doing so will not make people thinner. Our focus on eliminating fat isn't helping our children. Instead, this society is making them less healthy—physically and, most especially, mentally—by teaching them to fear fat.

I would argue that American society's approach to fat children is actually the abusive situation. Fat children receive the message daily that they are unworthy and unlovable. When the Safe School Improvement Act of 2010 (S.3739) was introduced, it did not include height and weight in the protected categories. This exclusion tells fat children that they are not worthy of being protected—that they deserve to be bullied. And these children are bullied often. A group of researchers out of the University of Michigan found that fat children experience bullying 63 percent more often than the average child. Fat children are not just bullied by other children at school—they are also bullied by family and other adults. Pattie Thomas argues this point on *Psychology Today*'s blog:

> Cruise any website that discusses weight and you will find a number of people who believe that telling a fat person they are less than human will encourage them to lose weight. People have said similar things in the comments for this blog. Stigma of fatness is not seen as a precursor to hate or bullying, but rather a duty on the part of authorities in order to correct what is obviously bad behavior. It is a cultural norm to believe that fat people are 100% responsible for their body shape and that they need to be motivated to change. Harassment is often seen as a motivation.

Our society repeatedly sends fat children the message that they do not deserve to be treated as other humans. This abuse of fat children is perhaps the most horrifying element of fat prejudice. That fat children are bullied by their peers is horrendous enough. The fact that parents, teachers, other adults and even the government feel like it is perfectly fine to torture and bully these children is detestable. And they do it all in the name of "health."

The worst part of the push toward eliminating fat children is that the very things we are doing to try and reduce fat are making our children fatter and less healthy. A study by Field et al. found that children who dieted tended to gain more weight than those that did not. In fact, the more I read studies about fat children, the more I believe that the younger a child diets, the more they may gain and the fatter they may get. Considering that mothers are being encouraged to limit children's intake in the womb (see "Perinatal Outcomes in Nutritionally Monitored Obese Pregnant Women: A Randomized Clinical Trial" for an example), such interventions could be creating *more* fat people, the thing these interventions are supposedly eliminating.

An article by journalist John Naish on the results of the Nazi-occupied Netherlands hunger winter noted that reducing food intake for pregnant mothers could be quite problematic:

> Some theories suggest that when a baby suffers malnutrition in the womb, a survival mechanism kicks in that pre-sets its metabolism in preparation for being born into a world of famine and starvation. This epigenetic alteration causes the body to give priority to fat storage over a developing robust liver, heart and brain.

So the very solutions presented for curing the childhood "obesity epidemic" are pretty much guaranteeing that the next generation will be bigger and less healthy than the current one!

This obsession with eliminating fat is also messing with children's relationship to food. The push toward "healthy" food and behavior can actually make children hate anything labeled "healthy." Humans have a tendency to rebel against things that are considered "good for us." In a study from 1998, Jennifer Orlet Fischer, Ph.D. and Leann Lipps Birch, Ph.D. found that restricting children's eating to healthy foods actually caused them to dislike such foods:

> Because parents tend to encourage children's consumption of fruits and vegetables and to limit foods high in energy, sugar, and fat, directive styles of child-feeding may negatively affect children's liking of these foods by teaching them to dislike the very foods we want them to consume and to prefer those that should be consumed in relatively limited quantities.

Some individuals in the Fatosphere found that the focus on weight loss often made them hate exercise and see it as punishment, rather than something to enjoy.

The things we are doing to try and make children lose weight may actually be backfiring, making them hate all things good for them. On top of that, our push towards eliminating fat children isn't making our children any smaller. However, it *is* increasing eating disorders tremendously.

I have often heard that our children are dying from Type 2 diabetes. However, as Linda Bacon argues, eating disorders are 229 times more prevalent in children than diabetes. In fact, as noted in Chapter 4, eating disorders and disordered eating are skyrocketing in children and are showing up in younger and younger children. This fear of the fat body can lead to death, considering that anorexia has the highest mortality rate of any mental illness, according to the National Alliance on Mental Illness (NAMI). Body dissatisfaction, not weight itself, increases suicide risks in girls, Rick Nauert, Ph.D. reports. So we are actually making our children mentally and physically less healthy by focusing on weight loss.

We are setting our children up to be even fatter adults, to hate exercise and healthy food, and to battle food issues for a lifetime while possibly facing the life-threatening diseases of anorexia and bulimia. As Lesley Kinzel notes on her blog *Two Whole Cakes:*

> By raising our kids to be obsessed with food, either the lack of it or the overabundance of it, we are stunting their development. We are holding them at the base of that pyramid instead of encouraging them to climb. No child should go hungry, ever, but nor should any child be made to feel stigmatized or guilty for eating. It does not work. It only produces kids who cannot fathom a world in which they will ever feel safe, and loved, and accepted, and real.

This push to eliminate "obesity" is only harming our children. We must stop abusing them in this way. If we are really interested in their health, why are we not teaching them about the HAES approach—a self-caring, loving and healthy way of life?

# Chapter 10
## It's Not About Health, It's About Medical Prejudice

**The problem is that doctors who see a fat person so often fail to** look beyond the fat, and not only fail to see nothing but the fat, but in the process deny treatment for whatever is actually wrong with you.

*Ann K. in a digital interview*

As noted before, fat individuals often receive the message from medical personnel that their bodies are wrong or broken, a fact that Ann K. pointed out in her interview, quoted above. A reminder from the section on prejudice: As many as 40 percent of physicians have a strong anti-fat bias. In fact, medical personnel repeatedly make the assumption that individuals are fat simply because they overeat and don't exercise.

In the Twitter thread #thingsfatpeoplearetold, which garnered hundreds of comments, ChironsGate noted a doctor asked, "How many frappuccinos do you drink a day?" after an incidence of unexplained rapid weight gain. This assumption that fat is the problem often leads the fat individual to suffer for no reason.

In fact, individuals in the Fatosphere experience so many difficult situations in dealing with the medical community that they created a blog just to discuss these medical atrocities. The blog *First, Do No Harm* allows fat individuals to email in stories of problems dealing with physicians, which Vesta44 then posts on the site. Story after story details everything from small incidences to life-threatening abuses that fat individuals experience at the hand of physicians.

The experiences include a pediatrician who ignored all the signs of anorexia because the patient had been "overweight" (Kitty) to the constant suggestion to try weight-loss surgery (Christine) to taking unneeded blood-pressure medicine (Jack) to having lactose intolerance blamed on being fat (Mareen) to having weight loss suggested as a cure for strep throat (Golda). HappyWriter details an excruciatingly painful process of seeing physician after physician to be told her weight was the problem again and again, even experiencing behavior meant to humiliate and shame her into losing weight. Eventually she was diagnosed with multiple sclerosis by a physician who took her symptoms seriously. She explains:

> I've had so much blamed on my weight, sometimes, I just prayed to get a doctor who would listen to me and see me as a person before they see the weight. I was finally diagnosed with MS, but I have to wonder—if it could've been caught earlier if I had a Dr who listened and [had] taken me seriously.

After a physician at Johns Hopkins refused to remove a cancerous tumor on her kidney because of her size, Suzy Smith had to choose another doctor, which delayed her surgery by two months.

These examples are just a few of the instances of medical fat prejudice I have heard about. I could probably fill a book with such instances.

Along the same lines, when dealing with mental health issues fat individuals can have everything blamed on their fat. As joannadeadwinter speaks of her experience:

Fat people get depressed because, well, fat people have feelings. I know that's a novel concept to many of my non-FA readers, but look at that! Whenever a visibly fat person walks into a helping professional's office and claims depression, it is likely she (I say "she" because women are especially victimized by this) will be asked what she is doing to fix her weight problem. The assumption, of course, is that fat people are depressed, universally, because of their weight. It does not occur to anyone that fat people could be depressed for the same reasons that so-called normal people are depressed—or, if a person's weight is the reason, that the problem is the stigma associated with her weight, not her weight in itself.

In fact, as Marilyn Wann noted in *The Fat Studies Reader*, "Mental health professionals are more likely to evaluate fat people negatively," a statement supported by research conducted by psychologists Gladys Agell and Esther D. Rothblum as well as sociologists Laura M. Young and Brian Powell.

These stories detail just a few of the experiences of fat prejudice by doctors floating around the Fatosphere.

Fat individuals experience oppression and prejudice when health professionals accuse them of lying about their diets and exercise amounts, an all-too-common occurrence. In a conversation on *The Rotund* entitled "On Disrespecting Doctors," Marshmallow told a frustrating experience about not being believed by a physician when seeking help for a foot injury. The physician told her to eat less and exercise—that that would solve the soreness in her foot. When she explained that she already exercised a great deal, the physician interrupted her, saying, "Don't take this the wrong way, but if you really did that much exercise? You would look very different now."

Even when fat individuals themselves are not accused of lying, their bodies are, says Anne Lutz in a digital interview:

> At my last appointment (to have a routine physical) the doctor took my blood pressure 4 times (it is naturally

low) then said that he didn't believe the results. When I mentioned that he had taken it four times, and that the nurse had taken it three, and asked him if his office was typically incompetent at taking blood pressure he backed off.

Fat individuals do receive the message that they are not honest about their habits. Once again, this bias is based in the belief that fat is caused by overeating and lack of exercise.

Physicians do experience a type of double-bind, however. They are often criticized for not recommending weight loss strategies to "obese" patients. For instance, a *Prev Med* article by psychologists J.L. Kristeller and R.A. Hoerr is critical of physicians who do not discuss "obesity" prevention with "obese" patients.

It is not surprising that physicians are hesitant to mention weight loss, however, since these recommendations usually fail, as do most attempts at weight loss (see previous discussion in Chapter 4), leading the physician often to see the patient as noncompliant, according to Roter and Hall. Additionally, fat individuals are less likely to return to a physician after such recommendations, a study by C.L. Olson, H.D. Schumaker and B.P. Yawn found.

So even if doctors see the ineffectiveness of encouraging weight loss, they are still expected to shame fat people into attempts at weight loss. This leads to a very ineffectual cycle: The doctor pushes weight loss. Fat individuals, usually having tried and failed to lose weight, go to the doctor less often. Then, when fat people die of something preventable, their fat is blamed. So doctors push weight loss.

The solution to such a cycle is to quit pushing weight loss.

I can't completely blame the physicians. From what I can find out, most medical schools do not teach even the possibility that a fat person can be healthy, or that fat can have protective qualities. In fact, I have spoken with a number of medical students who were about to enter residency. None of them had ever even heard of the "obesity paradox," let alone the protective qualities of fat. In fact, The Rudd Center for Food Policy and Obesity did a study and found that physicians who are given the full range of information have a tendency to be less prejudiced. However, as a negative from the Rudd Center's viewpoint—but not from mine—the Rudd Center researchers pointed out that such informed physicians are also less likely to suggest weight loss.

So doctors tend to just quote the status quo. They are just repeating what they have been told. They are just perpetuating a society-wide prejudice. And yet as a whole, the medical field and its supporting components are behind our current focus on "obesity."

As fat professional dancer Ragen Chastain says, "Somehow we've forgotten that body size is NOT a diagnosis."

Until the medical establishment faces the harm it has done—and continues to do—by trying to eradicate fat, we will continue to see prejudice in the medical field.

# Chapter 11
## So, If It's Not About Health, How Can We Get Healthier?

**Weight loss isn't the same as healthy habits, thin isn't the same** as healthy, and loving your body will never steer you wrong.

*Ragen Chastain on the blog* Dances With Fat

At this point, I have established that the push for weight reduction in our society is not about health. So if we really do want to get healthier, what do we do? The HAES model is one option that has found success both in scholarly research projects and among fat acceptance. We have so bought into the "obesity epidemic" that as a culture—especially including our medical establishment—we have been unwilling to consider other ways of thinking than the dieting mentality. To truly consider improving health, we must consider other paradigms than the thin-equals-healthy one that is so touted in our cultural rhetoric. The HAES paradigm is a different way of thinking about health, a new way of approaching both our behavior and our thinking about our bodies.

Defining the HAES approach can be a bit of a challenge. Bacon provides a definition that appears to be the overall accepted point of view of most HAES practitioners:

- Accepting and respecting the natural diversity of body sizes and shapes.

- Eating in a flexible manner that values pleasure and honors internal cues of hunger, satiety, and appetite.

- Finding the joy in moving one's body and becoming more physically vital.

For another view, there is guest blogger and nutritionist Deborah Kauffmann's definition on *The F-Word*:

> HAES is an approach to health and healthcare that promotes acceptance of natural body weight and an understanding that people come in all shapes and sizes. The HAES approach supports pleasurable and healthful eating that is based on internal cues of hunger and fullness as well as joyful movement.

Though on the surface HAES practices can closely resemble intentional weight loss behavior, there is one large difference—the end goal. HAES is "based on the simple premise that the best way to improve health is to honor your body," Bacon writes, whereas weight loss behaviors are only considered successful if the dieter loses and maintains a loss of weight. Bacon argues that rather than attempting weight loss, people should allow their bodies to settle at a natural set point. Basically, with the HAES philosophy, a person attempts to pay attention to their bodies' needs (for food, for rest, for exercise) while allowing the body to settle at a weight natural for that particular body.

The HAES model has been proven to improve both health indicators and self esteem. In a study comparing a set of women who dieted versus another set who practiced the HAES approach, the researchers found that those individuals who practiced HAES maintained long-term behavioral changes, whereas those who followed the dieting approach did not. Additionally, "reduction in dieting behavior, and heightened awareness and response to body signals resulted in improved health risk indicators for obese women."

Along similar lines, some studies have been done on intuitive eating, an aspect of the HAES approach that includes "eating in a flexible manner that values pleasure and honors internal cues of hunger, satiety, and appetite." A study of college-age girls and intuitive eating noted that body acceptance leads to intuitive eating:

> General unconditional acceptance predicted body acceptance by others, body acceptance by others predicted an emphasis on body function over appearance, body acceptance by others and an emphasis on body function predicted body appreciation, and an emphasis on body function and body appreciation predicted intuitive eating.

For the most part, the fat acceptance movement and the Fatosphere have embraced the HAES perspective, though there is some controversy surrounding this.

But what exactly does HAES mean to a fat person's daily living? Blogger Fillyjonk explained how she sees the HAES model:

> Anyone who's read Fatosphere blogs for any length of time will tell you that we are huge proponents of nutritious eating and regular movement, though for their own sake rather than for weight loss. Even the people who aren't all-HAES-all-the-time are interested in encouraging people to *normalize* their relationship with food—to stop seeing it as a source of sin or fear or love or comfort, not to turn around and make gluttony the main focus of our lives.

She also emphasizes that the HAES approach means "to care about your health MORE than you care about your weight, to care about your health independent of caring about your weight," which "takes vigilance." Kauffman states that practicing HAES "just means taking care of ourselves without focusing on weight loss," which appears to be the overall attitude towards the HAES model in the Fatosphere and fat acceptance movement as a whole.

Fat individuals who practice the HAES approach often feel healthier, and can be healthier according to medical standards, than those who diet. According to Bacon's study on the HAES model versus dieting, the HAES approach as a longer term positive outcome on health than does dieting, improving health indicators (blood sugar, blood pressure, heart rate, cholesterol) for a longer period of time.

When Kate Harding attacked diets that masquerade under terms such as "lifestyle change" or "a whole new way of eating," saying that such behavior changes didn't lead to weight loss either, blog commenter Louise felt like this post took away her hope of permanent weight loss:

> I've been putting the hard work into changing my habits for two years, slowly getting healthier, losing weight, and being thrilled by the benefits. Your post depresses me horribly. I rather wish I hadn't found your blog.

Responses to this comment help clarify that feeling good is an emphasis of the HAES approach. Blogger Sweetmachine responded to Louise by highlighting that feeling good is enough of a reward for eating better, while fillyjonk explained that success in HAES terms is more consistent than dieting:

> Plus, that way you actually get to appreciate your healthiness and good feelings. If you're too focused on weight loss, on days when the scale goes up you feel crappy— even if you should be feeling nourished by your healthy foods and energized by your workouts. If you stop measuring your success and self-worth by numbers, you get to enjoy your real successes a lot more.

Fatosphere participants found that by focusing on how they feel rather than on weight loss, they feel healthier and more accomplished following the HAES principles.

The HAES paradigm, though seemingly simple, can be hard to put into practice. Members of the fat acceptance community and the Fatosphere often struggle with the differences or lack of differences between the HAES approach and dieting. This dilemma is illustrated in a *Shapely Prose* blog conversation on diets not working. Discussing her exercise habits, Entangled made the following comment:

> I am trying to fight, but I lost a significant (though in reality not that large) amount of weight over the past two years. Mostly because I decided I was going to teach myself to run. I didn't really change my eating habits (beyond stopping when full, not stuffed), but I got SERIOUSLY, DEPRESSINGLY, OBSESSIVELY anal about them.
>
> On the days on which I concentrate on my habits—the fact that I can now run five miles, that I finished my first 5K in under 32 minutes, that my intense intervals are upwards of 7.5 mph—I feel great. When I concentrate on the visual results of those efforts, I feel like crap. Terrified that things will change, depressed that it matters, obsessive about food again.

She thought her comment might be "teetering towards diet-talk." Blogger Harding responded positively, explaining how she saw diet-talk:

> the diet talk I prohibit is the "Just do X and you'll lose the weight, and you'll feel better because you LOST WEIGHT!" Your comment, as I see it, was Health at Every Size talk. :)

This difference between HAES-talk and diet-talk reflects another discussion that pops up on the Fatosphere—the fact that some individuals will lose weight when practicing HAES behaviors. Commenter Caseyatthebat explains that she experienced "some weird internal reverse-size acceptance" because of losing weight:

> I tell myself that I will eat healthfully, move my body in a joyful way and accept the result, but in my head the "result" should be no weight loss, and I'm having a hard time accepting that, for me, it might mean some weight loss.

When discussing fantasies of thinness, commenter Mizerychik explained that she was one of the five percent of those who lost weight and kept it off for more than five years, which made her feel like she didn't belong in the Fatosphere or the fat acceptance community:

> I'm one of the 5%, and since reading more and more of the body acceptance movement, I kind of hate myself for it. Sometimes I feel like a traitor for reading this blog or that I don't belong, like I shouldn't comment because I am that freak of nature that often gets mentioned.

Members of the Fatosphere responded by emphasizing acceptance. Commenter Phledge responded by saying "don't feel bad about that," emphasizing that mizerychik's body was meant to be that way, while Meowser took the opportunity to expound on the philosophy behind the HAES approach:

> "Anti-dieting" does not equal "stay fat at all costs so you'll fit in with the rest of us fatasses." You, mizerychik, are a perfect illustration of what I'm talking about when I say, if you're truly meant to be a lot smaller than you are (or were), there's nothing I or anyone else can possibly do to stop you.

In her interview, Mustardseed puts it succinctly when she explains that the HAES perspective includes "accepting healthy thinness as well if that's what comes naturally." The differences between the HAES approach and dieting can be confusing because many of the tenets appear to be the same—however, as these conversations and comments show, the motivation behind them tends to be different.

From the outside, the Health At Every Size approach can be seen as a form of hedonism. Blogger fillyjonk explains her experience with common responses to the HAES perspective (emphasis in the original):

> But we're constantly being reviled—or at least treated with suspicion—for pimping overindulgence and inactivity. Why? Because we advocate treating yourself well, and that gets people's Puritan hackles up. Treating yourself well—doesn't that mean engaging in *constant sinnery?* Things that are good for you are supposed to feel like constant punishment, so if you're not punishing yourself, how can you ever do yourself good?

Exercise, especially, can be seen as a required punishment in the dieting mindset. However, self-care is actually incredibly hard, particularly for mothers or other caretakers. Self-care takes time, energy and effort—things we don't tend to have an excess of in our society. And it can feel selfish and self-centered.

Self-care actually isn't a selfish act, however. Rather, self-care is more like putting on your oxygen mask first in an emergency situation before trying to help others with theirs, as flight attendants stress in their pre-flight safety spiels. If we take care of ourselves, we then have the resources to help others, if we so choose. Yet often when a person finally starts taking care of themselves—especially someone who may have been overly caretaking in the past—they will be accused of selfishness. The HAES approach to well-being isn't hedonism or selfishness. The HAES approach is simply taking care of yourself the best way you can.

I often get asked about those who are "super-obese," "obese" to the point that fat causes problems. "Shouldn't they try to lose weight?" people often ask me. The answer for those individuals is still "no." Ask any of them to chart their diet history. I have yet to meet one who has not been on many, many diets. Chances are that at least part of the reason they are that fat has been attempts at weight loss. Even for these individuals, the HAES approach can be the answer. Since the HAES model encourages exercise and eating well no matter the situation, HAES practices can improve even these individuals' lives.

A study by Australian researchers led by P. Sumithran showed that low-calorie dieting can affect hormone levels long-term, causing an increase in appetite and a decrease in metabolism, leading to weight gain even on a maintenance regime. Pattie Thomas has addressed the problem of individuals who cannot carry their own weight when discussing a debate between psychologist John Foreyt and Linda Bacon:

> The question of mobility always comes up often when discussing the small portion of the population called the "super obese." I would argue the answer to mobility problems also does not lie in weight loss (especially since weight loss often weakens an already weak body). Not being able to carry one's weight is a problem that happens at all sizes. It is one of the criteria for what is known as frailty. I think two things would happen if we concentrated on health not weight. First, there would be fewer people at the higher end of the scale who had mobility problems because there would be places that would be safe (I'm speaking both socially and mechanically) for larger folk to exercise and develop the strength to carry their weight and I believe that if someone finds herself or himself in the condition of limited mobility, strength training would be the course of treatment, not weight loss. This is exactly the course of treatment for those at the lower end of the scale who become too weak to carry their weight.

So what we want to do rather than encourage weight loss

is to encourage exercise. This means making safe (both physically and psychologically) spaces and places for fat individuals to exercise. The HAES model is still the solution, even for fat individuals at the high end of the scale.

For those who are fat and do have illnesses, it can seem like the HAES approach is beyond their reach. And yet, argues Thomas, those who are fat and sick should be heading up the fight for the HAES paradigm:

> If I really believe in the principles of Health at Every Size®, then someone like me is on the front lines of these ideas. Someone like me is the one who has to fight for medical care that puts my health first rather than my weight. Someone like me has to speak out and say, it is not about weight, it is about health.

The HAES model can improve individuals' health, even if it does not cure or fix them. Because the HAES approach is adjustable for each individual, individuals with health challenges can use the principles of HAES to work within their own situations.

For instance, wellroundedtype2 had to adjust her diet because of diabetes. In a post on *Angry Grey Rainbows*, she says, "We all have a right to experiment with what works best for us, helps us to feel calm, to help manage our lives, to provide us with energy, to be healthy by our own definition—if that is something that matters to us."

So even if an individual has food allergies or diet restrictions, the HAES approach will work for them. Some individuals with physical limitations cannot exercise or must severely modify exercise. Yet the HAES principles encourage an individual to do what they can and not stress about what they cannot do.

Any individual can practice the HAES approach, even those with limitations, and receive benefits from such practices.

The HAES paradigm is a solution that many members of the Fatosphere and fat acceptance have found to heal their past unhealthy relationships with food and their bodies. Practicing the HAES approach is an action that shows both love for the body and love for the self. Though some controversy appears in the Fatosphere over exactly what the HAES approach means in daily life, how it is different from dieting, and how individuals with eating disorders deal with the HAES perspective, it appears to be working for many members of the Fatosphere and the fat acceptance community.

We keep trying to find a "one size fits all" solution to health, and we keep failing. We have seen from earlier chapters that we may not be able to trust studies. Physicians have bought into the myths, so we may not be able to trust them. What are we supposed to do?

I believe the solution, one the HAES paradigm embodies, is to trust yourself—trust your own body and your own experiences. Experiment. Experiment with food. Experiment with exercise. Experiment with new ways of thinking. What makes you feel better? What gives you more energy or less? What helps you feel healthier? What works FOR YOU?

We have been taught for so long that we cannot trust our bodies. Those who practice the HAES approach have found the opposite to be true—when we choose to trust our bodies, they will tell us exactly what they need. In a letter arguing against a *Biggest Loser* scenario at her school's rec center, fat studies scholar Cat Pausé said, "HAES does not argue that every size is healthy for every body, but that every body, regardless of size, can engage in healthy behaviours." When an individual starts practicing the HAES approach, they may find that their weight drops a little or goes up a little, though most remain the same, Linda Bacon found. What does happen, however, is that the vast majority of people feel better physically and have a better sense of self-esteem.

Will the HAES approach make everyone "healthy"? No, it won't. Will the HAES approach make everyone healthier? Yes, it will. And it makes many people happier as well. Given the failure of weight loss attempts in making anyone healthier in the long run, why don't we at least give it a try?

# Healthy Relationships with Food

AT THIS TIME, BECAUSE OF OUR FOCUS ON WEIGHT LOSS THE American people have a really screwed up relationship with food on the whole. Our media has in turn demonized everything from high fructose corn syrup to eggs. Our eating is filled with guilt and rebellion. The common theme in our society seems to be either eat low-fat, low carb, chemical-filled food and feel righteous, or eat good-tasting food and feel guilty. As a result, a person can see vegetables and fruit as punishment and junk food as a treat. As Marianne Kirby said on *The Rotund,* "I forgot how much worse vegetables taste when coated in guilt and obligation sauce."

Individuals in American society have forgotten how to feed themselves. Americans tend to live by food rules and the most current trend in diets.

When we let go of this idea of good food/bad food, a person can find a much healthier relationship with eating. Many individuals who practice the HAES approach report that when fruits and vegetables quit being "good," they enjoy them much more without the moral connections, as Kirby notes above. At the same time, when junk food is no longer forbidden people find that it no longer tastes quite so good. As Kate Harding has noted, "nothing's so attractive as the forbidden. If HAES ever catches on, people might start to notice that a great deal of junk food tastes like ass."

I think much of the focus on junk food comes from rebellion to our focus on "healthy" foods. Companies seem to recognize this, considering that Nestle bought the diet company Jenny Craig, as noted in Chapter 6.

Hirschmann and Munter also argue that the idea of "good" foods and "bad" foods actually causes people to binge on forbidden foods, and that when they legalize all foods, individuals tend to choose more nutrient-rich options.

This idea that we can trust our own body's signals—called "demand feeding," "intuitive eating," "attuned eating" and "mindful eating"—can be terrifying at first, especially for those who used to diet. Dieting teaches us to ignore our bodies' signals. To truly have a healthy relationship with food, we must be very aware of how our bodies feel about food. We must learn what hunger means, what fullness means, and to tell how food makes us feel.

If you are like me and spent 30 years ignoring all those signals, this can be a challenge. On my own journey, I was so out of touch with my body that I spent months learning to tell when I was hungry and full.

On Harding's post about devouring the world, Meg Thorton explained the challenge of demand feeding:

> Demand feeding was one of the hardest things for me to learn, and I'm still learning more about it every day. I've had to learn what it feels like to be hungry, had to learn what I do and don't want when I'm hungry, had to learn the difference between my stomach actually needing food, and me wanting something in my mouth because I'm feeling bored, nervous, upset, miserable, or just stuck for something to do.

Intuitive eating can be a very hard process to learn, but I have found the process worth it. Today I know how to feed my body what it wants, when it wants it. After years of being clueless how my body felt, I am now very aware of how much to eat and what to eat to make my body happy.

Of course, when a person first starts practicing intuitive eating, especially after years of dieting, they can be fearful of "devouring the world," as Kate Harding noted in a blog post that struck a chord for many people on the Fatosphere. Harding says that "*really* eating whatever we want…can be overwhelming and frankly frightening" (emphasis in the original). She goes on to note the power of that fear:

> But to really embrace demand feeding, I have to face that fear. I know, intellectually, that my fear is unfounded. I cannot possibly eat my own weight in Little Debbie oatmeal cream pies. I *know* it, but I still don't *believe* it.

People in our society, in particular women in our society, have been taught that we must control our urges—that if we allow ourselves to eat whatever we want, we will be out of control. Our society is terrified that we cannot be trusted, and in return we have a tendency not to trust our own bodies. Yet people who practice the HAES approach find that they and their bodies can be trusted to feed themselves well.

When starting intuitive eating individuals often find they are out of control, eating all those formerly forbidden foods. Hirschmann and Munter discuss this approach in their book *When Women Stop Hating Their Bodies.* These counselors who work with compulsive overeaters argue that by taking the idea of "good" or "bad" out of food, individuals are more likely to eat reasonable amounts:

> *Everyone* is terrified of losing control—of the gorging they believe will follow legalizing all food. They discover, however, that when they surround themselves with the foods they love *and* stop yelling at themselves for eating it, their cravings begin to diminish almost immediately. (emphasis in the original)

In fact, Harding also says that the best way to get over the fear of eating the world is to try and do so:

> So it makes a lot of sense that maybe the best way to stop feeling as if you're going to devour the WORLD is to

actually go ahead and *try* to devour the world. Because the first thing you'll realize is that you can't. And the next thing you'll realize is that you don't really want to. And once you get to that point, you might actually have a prayer of understanding your own internal hunger cues.

Most people who try to practice intuitive eating note that it can be a struggle at first. Chronic dieters are often so out of touch with their bodies that it can take awhile to adjust to paying attention to physical cues. For some individuals, figuring out what they want to eat can be quite a challenge. For others, learning what it means to feel full can be a process. However, many individuals find that issues with overeating or binging reduce or go completely away as they practice feeding their bodies intuitively.

Learning to trust your body can be tricky and sometimes complicated. In her book *Health At Every Size*, Linda Bacon says we can't trust cravings. I'm going to agree and disagree with her. I don't think we can trust cravings to tell us the truth, but in my own experience they do indicate that *something* is going on.

For instance, certain physical problems can cause cravings for high carbohydrate, high fat or junk foods. I have had issues with atypical Graves Disease. When I am not on meds I can crave high carbohydrate foods, a noted side effect of hyperthyroidism. Particular cravings can also indicate a lack of some nutritional element. If you crave particular foods, you might search the web for their nutritional content (yes, even most junk food has some nutritional content). It may be that your body is used to getting a nutrient from a particular food and will actually do better with other foods (though you have to teach it that) or supplements.

An example: I crave chocolate when I need copper. However, my body does better when I take copper supplements rather than eat large amounts of chocolate. As Liat from the blog *The*

*Spirit of Fat Acceptance* notes:

> [Cravings] tell me something is going on, but not always what. A great example: I kept craving Sweet Tarts. I could eat as many as I wanted and the craving was still there. If I ate a kiwi or an orange, however, the craving went away. I finally figured out that I was craving Vitamin C since I used to take a Vit C pill that tasted like Sweet Tarts. So, my body wasn't craving what I thought it was, but it did need something.

So cravings can be signals that something isn't right, though we can't trust the craving to tell us exactly what is going wrong.

Our society, as a whole, has unhealthy attitudes toward food and has wrapped so much morality around eating. Intuitive eating takes morality and its companion, rebellion, out of the situation, allowing people to learn how to feed their bodies in physically and emotionally beneficial ways.

Our society is eating disordered, but as individuals we do not have to be.

## *Attitude & Mental Health*

WHEN WE PRACTICE THE HAES PHILOSOPHY, WE CAN'T forget that any idea of overall health should include mental health. At times pressuring ourselves do the intuitive eating and exercise parts of the HAES approach can actually backfire—causing stress on the body and hurting health instead of improving it. Sometimes individuals can think that they must follow the HAES model religiously, approaching it with almost a diet mentality. For some people, focusing on nutrition and exercise in any way is likely to trigger old eating disorders or disordered eating. We must remember that balance is important in life; our physical, emotional and mental selves are all vital in the search for health.

I have heard a number of people in the Fatosphere comment that they must put their mental health before worrying about nutrition and exercise. Deeleigh (Deidre Calarco) of *Big Fat Blog* notes:

> To me, thinking that you can fail or do badly at HAES is a misinterpretation of HAES. Mental health is the foundation of HAES. Some former dieters are never going to feel comfortable with any eating rules whatsoever (Regular meal times? Vegetarianism? No way.) or with any amount of formally organized movement.

Of course, society appears to expect fat people to focus on our physical health above all else, especially after rejecting the need for smaller bodies. Yet proponents of the HAES model find that balance is a requirement for a healthy life. Deeleigh explains the balance of the HAES perspective so very well:

> At the core, HAES isn't about following a conventionally "healthy" way of eating, or about being physically active. HAES is about thinking about these issues and deciding, as an independent and self aware adult, what feels best to you and how to live your life. It's about treating yourself with compassion, and about understanding, forgiving, and making room for your limitations. It is never about guilt or about being good or bad.

Along with these words, Dee provided an excellent graphic to explain the balance required behind the HAES perspective:

## HEALTH AT EVERY SIZE

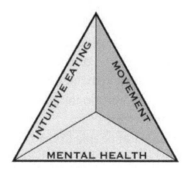

Without the foundation of mental health, our physical health can crumble.

As I have experienced my own journey using the HAES philosophy and as I have read the experiences of others on the Fatosphere, I think that the HAES model is a process rather than an event. For some long-time dieters, ALL attempts at "healthy" behavior must go out the window for a time. This rebellion can be a time to explore formerly forbidden foods, as Hirschmann and Munter call foods previously labeled "bad," can be a time to reject exercise, and can be a time to discard all the previous rules. Though many people in our society will have a conniption fit at such behavior, this rebellion can be a vital part of the process. After a short period of hedonistic behavior, most individuals find that such behavior simply doesn't feel good and will start exploring food and exercise habits that do feel good—leading to better mental, emotional and physical health in the end.

An important part of the HAES model is our own attitudes toward our bodies and our selves. Our mental health and state of mind is as important as our physical bodies. After years and years of failed diets, many of us crawl to fat acceptance feeling like failures, having disappointed ourselves and others time after time. Allowing ourselves to be "bad," to rebel from the diet mentality, can free us from all those old unrealistic expectations.

On top of that, choosing to love our bodies and ourselves can be a healing process in itself. Personally, I believe that a positive attitude toward my body can actually aid in healing any physical issues that might be present, a belief supported by experts such as psychologist Oakley Ray of Vanderbilt University, on top of simply making life more enjoyable. The HAES approach is about relaxing, giving up the "shoulds" that we have lived with so long. And better health is only achieved through the health of the whole person—mental health included.

# Finding Support

ONE OF THE KEYS TO SURVIVING BEING FAT IN A FAT-HATING world is to find a support group. We need a place to go where we can feel safe and people to talk to who understand. We need to hear how others have survived our particular situation. Our scientific and medical communities focus on statistics and on what works for the majority. However, what if my body doesn't work like the majority of other peoples' bodies do? One of the wonderful things about support groups is that people share what has worked for them, even if it is out of the norm. The participant can decide what to try and what to leave alone.

Another plus for support groups is that sometimes such groups motivate individuals to try behaviors or activities they would be unwilling to try or think themselves incapable of trying on their own. As Ragen Chastain says:

> And a concept that I learned long ago in a psychology class came to mind—the idea that if you see a single person do something it suddenly becomes possible to you. I think that this is particularly important in a society where we're told repeatedly (by industries who are trying to sell us stuff) that as fat people we're practically immobile.

In fact, many members of the Fatosphere have made comments to that effect. Fatosphere participants have noted being encouraged to try exercise in types or ways that they have not before. Additionally, individuals are encouraged to try eating in new and different ways. Members have also shared how they have worked through body image and self-esteem issues. Such support can help individuals improve their lives and health in many different ways.

Support for the fat individual exists in real life as well. Active fat liberation communities exist in New York City and San

Francisco. Some other large cities may have gatherings as well. For those of us who do not have access to these groups, we can find support online in the Fatosphere.

To conclude this section on the HAES model—in my experience, most people who say they want to lose weight for their health just want to lose weight. If it is really about health, how about trying the HAES approach? The HAES approach has been proven to improve health no matter where you start out.

If you are in that place of thinking that your health sucks because of your weight, I feel for you. If you need to try one more diet, do. If you can, keep reading fat acceptance stuff while you diet. If you can't, come back if it does not work. If you are thinking about some kind of weight loss surgery, I encourage you to throw yourself into the HAES approach and fat acceptance for one year—just one year. Give it the best try you can. If it doesn't work for you, go have the surgery next year.

But in my experience, the HAES model works, and works well.

# Chapter 12
## If It's Not About Health, How Can Fat People Get Good Health Care?

**Many fat individuals have found that when dealing with the medical** industry it takes a great deal of assertive behavior to obtain good health care. For instance, fat individuals often "get a diet, rather than a diagnosis" when dealing with the medical community, Marilyn Wann notes in her book *Fat!So?*. In an online interview with car, a common commenter in the Fatosphere, car expressed frustration at physicians' stubborn refusal to accept the scientific evidence that fat does not immediately equal a health risk. "The 'easy' answer is still that fat is bad and unhealthy," she said, "and it seems that stories that show it's not that simple are just buried."

In order to resist fat bias, fat individuals must learn to transverse cultural, medical and scientific rhetoric—often learning to formulate science-based arguments just to receive basic necessities like health care. In a post on *Shapely Prose*, Piper argues on "how important it is as a fat person to arm yourself with knowledge" when dealing with doctors.

A common technique used by some individuals in the

Fatosphere when dealing with physicians is to send a letter to a new doctor. The original text of one commonly used letter came from Hanne Blank and can be borrowed from her blog (see www.cat-and-dragon.com/stef/fat/hanne.html). The letter introduces the fat individual and explains the individual's boundaries and requirements regarding weight. Blog commenter Sticky did much the same thing in person:

> When I met with the new doctor for the first time, I immediately launched into a speech about how I don't need diet advice, need her to treat me beyond weight, blah blah. I ended it with asking if she felt she could treat me without focusing on my weight. She said yes, and that was that. I was very nervous and teary about it though. I even wrote a few things down to say.

On *Shapely Prose,* blog commenter JupiterPluvius has no problem with saying "This appointment is over. I need to leave now."

One fat acceptance community member, Stef, maintains a fat friendly health care professional list (found at http://cat-and-dragon.com/stef/fat/ffp.html) that allows people to find health care professionals who will treat them without making an issue of their weight.

Fat individuals have a number of different techniques that assist them in getting good health care. Fat individuals on their own often find they cannot learn enough to combat the might of the medical community. However, with the resources, knowledge and support of the Fatosphere, these individuals can find the information and support needed to get good health care.

In order to refute the standard medical dogma, bloggers often take common assumptions about fat or anything in the media dealing with fat—a research study, a newspaper article, an online posting, or an advertisement—and examine such ideas and conclusions together with their readers. The members of the community examine the wording, the research methods, and the conclusions of such artifacts looking for flaws, fallacies or legitimacy within them. They will quickly point out any obvious or hidden fat prejudice within the pieces. Together, then, the community will come to an understanding of the relevance of data or lack of legitimacy within the piece, slowly building an accepted core of knowledge that the community agrees upon.

In an excellent example of this, the Fatosphere closely examined a study of the Amish that concluded that genetic predisposition to fat could be overcome by exercise. The authors of the study, Evadnie Rampersaud, Ph.D. and colleagues, argued that genetically fat individuals could stay thin by participating in "about 3 to 4 hours of moderately intensive physical activity, such as brisk walking, house cleaning, or gardening" a day. In a post on the blog *Fatistician,* Shinobi42 asserted that it is unrealistic to expect the average American to live like the Amish. In posts on their own blogs, bloggers Bronwen and April D both emphasized that expecting an individual to exercise 3-4 hours a day is not realistic.

On the blog *A Day in the Fat Life,* Bronwen argued that such extreme measures were not feasible: 'So, now, besides eating a starvation diet, I also have to exercise for four hours a day? Ummmm, in what universe is that really a viable solution?" On a post entitled "Better Things I Could Do With the Time," April D provided a list of other things she could do with the time, including belly dancing and doing her homework.

Bloggers also questioned how the results would be spun in the media. Blogger Living 400 lbs argued that the study was not about weight loss, but that the media would portray it with that spin anyway. "Yeah, whatever you do," Shinobi42 said, "don't interpret this study to mean anything about how it might be unrealistic to expect every person on earth to be thin while living a modern lifestyle." Blogger Sandy Szwarc at *Junk-*

*food Science* explains problems with the study itself:

> Despite the great import being given this study's find-
> ings as a prescription for weight management, a prudent
> precaution is to remember that it was an epidemiological
> data dredge study. Anytime we throw enough variables
> into a computer, it's bound to find some *correlations*, but
> that doesn't mean they mean anything. This study is no
> different.

Together, members of the Fatosphere have come to understand both the relevance of the data and the implications of
such a study.

As another example, fat individuals have learned to gather
fat-supportive facts and present them to health care professionals as an argument for good care. The community at *Big Fat
Blog* put together a fact sheet, called "Big Fat Facts," on weight
loss and fat health from a fat acceptance point of view (www.
bigfatfacts.com/).

Together, individuals in the Fatosphere are learning to rein-
terpret the dominant rhetoric in a more fat-friendly light.

I have shown that we pretty much can't trust the science
behind fat. In fact, I encourage you not to take my word for it.
Rather, I encourage you to experiment in your own life. Has
dieting worked for you? Have you kept lost weight off? Have
you liked yourself more? Three years after a diet, do you feel
better or worse physically? How about better or worse about
yourself?

If you are reading this book, you are probably tired of the
failure of dieting. So why not try the HAES perspective? Why
not try being gentle and loving with your body, rather than
trying to force it into a mold it was never meant for? Why not
try working with your body instead of against it?

If you are a medical professional, has encouraging weight
loss made your patients better in the long run? If not, why not
tell them about the HAES approach and see if they are more

likely to comply? If bugging them to lose weight has failed, why not try something new and different?

What we have done in the past hasn't worked, so why keep doing it?

I have found I must take responsibility for my own health and become my own researcher. Though my physician may be an expert in medicine, I have become an expert on my own body. And I only work with medical professionals who respect that fact. I expect a physician to take my experience into account when approaching medical solutions.

We have to pay attention to how our own individual bodies react and function, and we have to make sure our medical professionals hear that experience.

# Chapter 13
# Health Intervention Failure, Rhetorical Success

"Everybody knows" fat is bad for you. "Everybody knows" that we are in an "obesity epidemic." "Everybody knows" that fat people are fat because they eat too much and exercise too little. "Everybody knows" that fat people will lose weight if they just exercise and eat less. Ask any general person on the street, and the chances are high that they will tout these messages. Everybody knows these things just like everybody knew the world was flat and that the sun revolved around the Earth. And just like the major shifts in thinking to see the world as round and the Earth as revolving around the sun, to change this thinking requires a paradigm shift. A shift away from focusing on weight loss is required for us to call ourselves a fair people and to actually make health a focus.

American cultural attitudes regarding "obesity" have created a situation in which prejudice and oppression have been legitimized by an ethos of scientific and medical rhetoric, language we are tempted to see as unbiased. By using science-based wording with specific negative connotations (such as the terms "epidemic" and "disease"), a sense of urgency—a moral panic—has been ignited within the population that, in turn, places the fat individual in the Sisyphean bind—a bind that the fat individual is not likely to escape without resisting the many negative messages about fat.

Medical rhetoric—acting as a form of bio-power and being used as a "control mechanism," in rhetorician Bernadette Longo's terms—is being used to try to normalize this marginalized population, in turn marginalizing them further. To combat this, fat individuals themselves must make a paradigm shift—understanding that fat is not bad, nor are they bad for being fat.

Medical research contains a very powerful ethos, a perceived credibility that has been used to reinforce the belief that fat is unhealthy. In turn, this belief that fat is unhealthy is being used to legitimize and support the oppression of fat individuals.

Fat individuals are continually fed the message to lose weight in order to avoid prejudice. However, fat people repeatedly find that weight loss attempts require time, energy and money and do not lead to permanent weight loss—in fact, they often lead to weight gain. This places the fat person in a frustrating cycle of gain and loss without solution, a Sisyphean bind. To add frustration to this cycle, though there exists dissension within the ranks of medical researchers, the dominant voice in the medical industry—the rhetoric that the average individual hears regularly—continues to perpetuate the belief that fat in itself is unhealthy, which in turn creates a hostile environment for the fat individuals.

As we have seen in this book, fat prejudice has been encouraged and legitimized by the medical and diet industries, industries with money to gain from futile attempts at weight loss. Dietitian and scholar Lucy Aphramor suggests that continuing to emphasize an approach—weight loss—that doesn't work and has been proven to have negative consequences is unethical and should be stopped.

Albert Einstein said that insanity is "doing the same thing over and over again and expecting different results." Weight loss dieting, even when you call it "a lifestyle change," has proven to be an insane option for most people. By continuing to empha-size weight loss, the medical community is going against their own Hippocratic oath to "first, do no harm." This practice is especially heinous since it perpetuates the very condition it is supposed to fix, leaving the fat person in a horrendous bind.

This quote from Linda Bacon on the ASDAH HAES blog argues for the real enemy:

> The real enemy, then, is not weight, but weight stigma. Fear of fat is much more harmful than actual adiposity, distracting us from true threats to our health and well-be-ing. Let's stop the demonization and switch our emphasis to Health At Every Size®, encouraging health-promoting behaviors for all.

So we need to quit focusing on weight loss and instead fo-cus on losing our negative attitudes about our own fat and fat people in general. We need to become accepting rather than judging.

When I learned the facts about "obesity," I grew very, very mad. For the first time in my life, I understood that I was not the problem—society is. I understood that all of those attempts at weight loss were just a way to get my money and make me hate myself. For the first time I understood that I didn't deserve to be oppressed or ridiculed.

I wrote this book so that some of you might understand that you are not the problem. I wrote this book in the hopes that we might change how medicine approaches health in the fat individual. I wrote this book to help change the paradigm.

It is my hope that the reader might heal in some way from this information—learning to love your own or another's fat body, recognizing the harm of focusing on weight loss as a technique to better health, realizing that whether or not you lose weight you can feel better. If you are fat, do not be sur-prised if this book makes you angry. That is part of the process.

I encourage you to learn more about health and fat and to seek to heal. You will find that you get healthier in body and mind in the process.

The push to reduce "obesity," couched in the terms of an epidemic, is a rhetorical success and a complete and total health intervention failure. This failure is understandable when we realize that weight loss is about everything but health. And yet people will fight tooth and nail to believe that weight loss attempts are about health. I have found again and again that when I try to tell them about the HAES paradigm, they reject the idea.

People don't want to get skinny to be healthier—that's just a smoke screen for our society's true wants: desirability, status, traditional beauty, and, for the truly fat, social acceptability. The push to reduce fat isn't about health—it's about everything but! Yet rhetorically, we are convinced that fat is the problem and the enemy.

By focusing on weight loss, all our society is doing is hurting the very people it is supposedly helping. Focusing on weight loss just shoves the fat individual into the Sisyphean bind. Focusing on weight loss hasn't worked. Focusing on weight loss has not made us one bit healthier.

It is time to shift the paradigm. Let's start focusing on what really makes people healthy—mentally, physically and socially. Let's focus on loving our bodies and practicing Health At Every Size.

# Notes

## Chapter 2

"...based on the Body Mass Index (BMI), which in itself is very controversial." For information on the controversy surrounding BMI, see the article "Increasing prevalence of overweight among US adults from *The National Health and Nutrition Examination Surveys*, 1960 to 1991" by Kuczmarski, Flegal, Capbell, & Johnson (1994).

"BMI is calculated by taking a person's weight and dividing it by the square of his or her height." For information on calculating BMI, see the article "Excess Deaths Associated With Underweight, Overweight, and Obesity" by Flegal, Graubard, Williamson, & Gail (2005).

"...since some pharmaceuticals cause weight gain..." Information on pharmaceuticals causing weight gain can be found within the article "Body Weight Changes Associated With Psychopharmacology" by Vanina, Podolskaya, Sedky, Shahab, Siddiqui, Munshi, & Lippmann (2002).

"...since depression can cause weight gain..." A look at depression causing weight gain can be found in B. Blaine's "Does Depression Cause Obesity?" (2008).

"...since illnesses such as hypothyroidism or Cushing's syndrome can cause weight gain..." Information on illness causing weight gain can be found through the Mayo Clinic (www.mayoclinic.com).

"Another study suggested that 'obesity' is caused by a virus..." The study stating that "obesity" is caused by a virus was written by Atkinson, Dhurandhar, Allison, Bowen, Israel, Albu, & Augustus (2005).

# Chapter 3

"Children as young as preschool age already have anti-fat bias..." Rich, Essery, Sanborn, DiMarco, Morales & LeClere examined children's attitudes toward weight in the journal *Obesity* (2008).

"As many as 25 percent of adolescents report weight-based teasing throughour their adolescent years by their peers..." "Logitudinal and secular trends in weight-related teasing during adolescence" was written by Haines et al. and published in the journal *Obesity* (2008).

"...with 'obese' adolescents reporting a signficantly higher incidence of teasing..." Data on teasing by peers and family can be found in Libbey et al.'s "Teasing, disordered eating behaviors, and psychological morbidities among overweight adolescents" published in the journal *Obesity* (2008).

"...younger individuals experience more denigration in relation to attractiveness." For stereotyping of "obese" individuals according to age, see Hebl, Ruggs, Singletary & Beal's 2008 article "Perceptions of obesity across the lifespan," published in the proceedings of the *20th Annual Meeting of the Association of Psychological Science.*

# Chapter 4

"...yet many fat individuals are that way because of genetics..." Studies that support genetics as the foundation for most individuals' weight include: A.J. Stunkard et al. (1986); A. J. Stunkard, J.R.Harris, N.L.Pederson, & G.E.McClearn (1990); and Wardle, Carnell, Haworth, & Plomin (2008).

# Chapter 5

"Studies exist concluding that diabetes is caused by fat..." For information on studies saying diabetes is caused by fat, see M.A. Lazar's 2005 article "How Obesity Causes Diabetes: Not a Tall Tale," which was published in the journal *Science*.

"...yet studies also exist arguing that diabetes causes fat." Studies arguing that diabetes causes fat include Sigal et al.'s "Acute Postchallenge Hyperinsulinemia Predicts Weight Gain: a Prospective Study" published in 1997 in the journal *Diabetes* and Yost, Jensen, & Eckel's 1995 article "Weight Regain Following Sustained Weight Reduction Is Predicted by Relative Insulin Sensitivity" published in *Obesity Research*.

"Studies exist that argue fat is a primary cause of heart disease..." Medical articles that argue for fat as a cause of heart disease include Eckel & Krauss's "American Heart Association Call to Action" published in *Circulation* (1998).

"A study suggests that gallbladder problems can even be caused by weight loss." The study showing that gallbladder issues can be caused by dieting was written by Shiffman et al. and published in *The American Journal of Gastroenterology* (2008).

"In these studies we can find that fat provides many positive aspects to health." The protective qualities of fat can be found in numerous studies:

- Romero-Corral et al.'s "Association of Bodyweight with Total Mortality and with Cardiovascular Events in Coronary Artery Disease: a Systematic Review of Cohort Studies," which was published in *Lancet* (2006);

- Kalantar-Zadeh et al.'s "Survival Advantages of Obesity in Dialysis Patients," which was published in *The American Journal of Clinical Nutrition* (2005);

- Donohoe et al.'s "Perioperative Evaluation of the Obese Patient" published in *The Journal of Clinical Anesthesia* (2011); Hutagalung et al.'s "The Obesity Paradox in Surgical Intensive Care Unit Patients," published in *The Journal of Intensive Care Medicine* (2011);

- Doehner et al.'s "Inverse relation of body weight and weight change with mortality and morbidity in patients with type 2 diabetes and cardiovascular co-morbidity: An analysis of the PROactive study population" published in *The International Journal of Cardiology* (2011);

- Sohn et al.'s "Obesity Paradox in Amputation Risk Among Nonelderly Diabetic Men" published in the journal *Obesity* (2012);

- Myers et al.'s "The Obesity Paradox and Weight Loss" published in *The American Journal of Medicine* (2011);

- Memtsoudis et al.'s "Mortality of Patients With Respiratory Insufficiency and Adult Respiratory Distress Syndrome After Surgery: The Obesity Paradox" published in *The Journal of Intensive Care Medicine* (2011);

- Lainscak et al.'s "Body Mass Index and Prognosis in Patients Hospitalized with Acute Exacerbation of Chronic Obstructive Pulmonary Disease" published in The *Journal of Cachexia, Sarcopenia and Muscle* (2011);

- Scherbakov et al.'s "Body Weight After Stroke: Lessons From the Obesity Paradox" published in the journal *Stroke* (2011);

- Ovbiagele et al.'s "Obesity and Recurrent Vascular Risk After a Recent Ischemic Stroke" published in the journal *Stroke* (2011); and

- Katsnelson et al.'s "Obesity Paradox and Stroke: Noticing the (Fat) Man Behind the Curtain" published in the journal *Stroke* (2011).

"Studies in Japan and Canada came to much the same conclusion as Flegal's team." Studies that reached the same conclusion as Flegal's team, that "overweight" individuals live the longest, include "BMI and All-Cause Mortality Among Japanese Older Adults: Findings from the Japan Collaborative Cohort Study" by Tamakoshi et al. (2010) and "Results From a National Longitudinal Study of Canadian Adults" by Orpana et al. (2010). Both articles were published in the journal *Obesity*.

"...increased cortisol levels increase blood sugar levels." For information on how cortisol increases blood sugar levels, see Khani and Tayek's "Cortisol Increases Gluconeogenesis in Humans: Its Role in the Metabolic Syndrome" (2001).

"We also know that continued stress will increase cortisol levels and that fat prejudice causes stress." See Meyerhoff, Oleshansky and Mougey's "Psychologic Stress Increases Plasma Levels of Prolactin, Cortisol, and POMC-Derived Peptides in Man" (1988) for a deeper look at how stress increases cortisol levels.

"We also know that continued stress will increase cortisol levels and that fat prejudice causes stress." Peter Muennig explores the relationship between fat prejudice and stress on the body in "the Body Politic: the Relationship Between Stigma and Obesity-Associated Disease" (2008).

"Low calorie dieting also increases cortisol levels." Tomiyama et al. found that low calorie dieting increased cortisol levels. This finding was published in "Low calorie dieting increases cortisol" within the journal *Psychosomatic Medicine* (2010).

"For instance, physicians are likely to spend less time with fat patients, and are less likely to order appropriate tests for fat patients, while ordering a number of unneeded tests." For more information on doctors and the testing of "obese" patients, see Østbye et al.'s article "Associations Between Obesity and Receipt of Screening Mammography, Papanicolaou Tests, and Influenza Vaccination: Results from the Health and Retirement Study (HRS) and the Asset and Health Dynamics Among the Oldest Old (AHEAD) Study" published in the *American Journal of Public Health* (2005) and Hebl & Xu's "Weighing the Care: Physicians' Reactions to the Size of a Patient" published in *The International Journal of Obesity* (2001).

# Suggested Reading Lists

## Fat Studies Books and Articles

Bacon, Linda. (2008). *Health At Every Size: The Surprising Truth About Your Weight.* Dallas, TX: Benbella Books, Inc.

Bacon, L., Stern, J. S., Loan, M. D. V., & Keim, N. L. (2005). Size acceptance and intuitive eating improve health for obese, female chronic dieters. *Journal of American Dietetic Association,* 105, 929-936.

Campos, P. F. (2004). *The Diet Myth: Why America's Obsession with Weight Is Hazardous to Your Health.* New York, NY: Penguin Group (USA), Inc.

Campos, P. F., Saguy, A., Ernsberger, P., Oliver, J. E., & Gaesser, G. A. (2006). The Epidemiology of Overweight and Obesity: Public Health Crisis or Moral Panic? *International Journal of Epidemiology,* 35(1), 55-60.

Fraser, L. (1997). *Losing It: America's Obsession with Weight and the Industry that Feeds on It.* New York, NY: Dutton Adult.

Gaesser, G. A. (1999). Thinness and Weight Loss: Beneficial or Detrimental to Longevity. *Medicine and Science in Sports and Exercise,* 31(8), 118-1128.

Gaesser, G. A. (2002). *Big Fat Lies: The Truth About Your Weight and Your Health.* Carlsbad, CA: Gurze Books.

Gaesser, G. A. (2003). Is It Necessary to Be Thin to Be Healthy? *Harvard Health Policy Review*, 4(2), 40-47.

Gard, M. (2005). *The Obesity Epidemic: Science, Morality and Ideology*. New York, NY: Routledge.

Harding, K., & Kirby, M. (2009*). Lessons from the Fat-o-sphere: Quit Dieting and Declare a Truce With Your Body.* New York, New York: Penguin Group (USA), Inc.

Hirschmann, J. R., & Munter, C. H. (1995). *When Women Stop Hating Their Bodies*. New York: Fawcett Books.

Kolata, G. (2007a). *Rethinking Thin: The New Science of Weight Loss—and the Myths and Realities of Dieting*. New York: Farrar, Straus, and Giroux.

Oliver, J. E. (2006a). *Fat Politics: The Real Story Behind America's Obesity Epidemic*. USA: Oxford University Press.

Oliver, J. E. (2006b). The Politics of Pathology: How Obesity Became an Epidemic Disease. *Perspectives in Biology and Medicine*, 49(4), 611-627.

Rothblum, E., and Solovay, S. (Eds.) (2009). *The Fat Studies Reader*. New York and London: New York University Press.

Saguy, A., and Ward, A. (2010). Coming Out as Fat: Rethinking Stigma. *Social Psychology Quarterly*, forthcoming.

Saguy, A. C., and Almeling, R. (2008). "Fat in the Fire? Science, the News Media, and the 'Obesity Epidemic.'" *Sociological Forum*, 23(1), 53-83.

Solovay, S. (2000). *Tipping the Scales of Justice: Fighting Weight-Based Discrimination*. New York: Prometheus Books.

Wann, M. (1999). *Fat!So? Because You Don't Have to Apologize for Your Size!* Berkeley, CA: Ten Speed Press.

# Fat Positive Internet Resources

*Big Fat Blog:* www.bigfatblog.com/

*Fat body politics* **tumblr:** http://fatbodypolitics.tumblr.com/

**Fat Positive/HAES Marketing Facebook group:**
http://www.facebook.com/groups/207243959295384/

**Fat Studies Facebook group:**
http://www.facebook.com/groups/5565108314/

**Linda Bacon, Ph.D.'s Health At Every Size community:**
http://haescommunity.org/

*Hey, fat chick!* **tumblr:** http://heyfatchick.tumblr.com/

**Kath Read's** *Fat Heffalump* **blog:**
http://fatheffalump.wordpress.com/

**Lara Frater's** *Fat Chicks Rule!* **blog:**
http://fatchicksrule.blogs.com/fat_chicks_rule/

**Linda Bacon's website:** http://www.lindabacon.org/

*Living ~400 lbs* **blog:** http://living400lbs.wordpress.com/

**Marianne Kirby's** *The Rotund* **blog:** http://therotund.com

**Ragen Chastain's** *Dances with Fat* **blog:**
http://danceswithfat.wordpress.com/

*The Well Rounded Mama* **blog:**
http://wellroundedmama.blogspot.com/

FOR UPDATED LINKS, SEE:
www.loniemcmichael.com/fatlinks

# About the Author

Lonie McMichael has wanted to be a writer since age 3. For many years she practiced her trade as a technical writer in the high tech industry. After going to graduate school, Lonie found her calling in fat studies, exploring the fat individual's experience. Graduating with a Ph.D. in technical communication and rhetoric, she wrote her dissertation on the medical rhetoric surrounding the "obesity epidemic" and how such rhetoric legitimizes fat prejudice—topics which have become two separate books, *Talking Fat* and *Acceptable Prejudice?* (the latter to be published by Pearlsong Press in 2013).

She is currently teaching professional and technical writing at the University of Colorado at Colorado Springs and working on her third book about things fat. Visit her on the web at www.loniemcmichael.com.

A BOOK GROUP STUDY GUIDE TO *TALKING FAT* CAN BE DOWN-loaded at www.pearlsong.com/talkingfat.htm.

# About Pearlsong Press

PEARLSONG PRESS IS AN INDEPENDENT publishing company dedicated to providing books and resources that entertain while expanding perspectives on the self and the world. The company was founded by Peggy Elam, Ph.D., a psychologist and journalist, in 2003.

We encourage you to enjoy other Pearlsong Press books, which you can purchase at www.pearlsong.com or your favorite bookstore. Keep up with us through our blog at www.pearlsongpress.com.

## FICTION:

*The Falstaff Vampire Files*—paranormal adventure by Lynne Murray
*Larger Than Death*—a Josephine Fuller mystery by Lynne Murray
*Large Target*—a Josephine Fuller mystery by Lynne Murray
*The Season of Lost Children*—a novel by Karen Blomain
*Fallen Embers* & *Blowing Embers*—Books 1 & 2 of The Embers Series,
paranormal romance by Lauri J Owen
*The Fat Lady Sings*—a young adult novel by Charlie Lovett
*Syd Arthur*—a novel by Ellen Frankel
*Bride of the Living Dead*—romantic comedy by Lynne Murray
*Measure By Measure*—a romantic romp with the fabulously fat by
Rebecca Fox & William Sherman
*FatLand*—a visionary novel by Frannie Zellman
*The Program*—a suspense novel by Charlie Lovett
*The Singing of Swans*—a novel about the Divine Feminine
by Mary Saracino

## ROMANCE NOVELS & SHORT STORIES FEATURING BIG BEAUTIFUL HEROINES:

by Pat Ballard, the Queen of Rubenesque Romances:
*Dangerous Love* | *The Best Man* | *Abigail's Revenge*
*Dangerous Curves Ahead: Short Stories* | *Wanted: One Groom*
*Nobody's Perfect* | *His Brother's Child* | *A Worthy Heir*
by Rebecca Brock—*The Giving Season*
& by Judy Bagshaw—*At Long Last, Love: A Collection*

HEALING THE WORLD ONE BOOK AT A TIME

Lightning Source UK Ltd.
Milton Keynes UK
UKHW010113280122
397829UK00003B/924